Treating Generalized Anxiety Disorder

Treating Generalized Anxiety Disorder

EVIDENCE-BASED STRATEGIES, TOOLS, AND TECHNIQUES

JAYNE L. RYGH and WILLIAM C. SANDERSON

THE GUILFORD PRESS
New York   London

Library of Congress Cataloging-in-Publication Data

Rygh, Jayne L.
  Treating generalized anxiety disorder : evidence-based strategies, tools, and techniques / Jayne L. Rygh, William C. Sanderson.
    p. cm.
  Includes bibliographical references and index.
  ISBN 1-59385-039-5 (pbk.: alk. paper)
   1. Anxiety—Handbooks, manuals, etc. 2. Cognitive therapy—Handbooks, manuals,
etc. I. Sanderson, William C. II. Title.
  RC531.R93 2004
  616.85′ 220651—dc22

                                                    2004009229

About the Authors

Jayne L. Rygh, PhD, is a senior psychologist at the Cognitive Therapy Center of New York, where she is both a psychotherapist and a supervisor. Using cognitive-behavioral and schema therapies, Dr. Rygh treats clients suffering primarily from anxiety, depressive, and personality disorders. In addition, she has served as an independent evaluator and research psychotherapist in numerous National Institute of Mental Health grants on the treatment of anxiety disorders.

William C. Sanderson, PhD, is Professor of Psychology at Hofstra University. He has served on numerous national committees, including the American Psychiatric Association's DSM-IV Anxiety Disorders Workgroup, and was recently Chair of the Committee on Science and Practice (a task force aimed at identifying and promoting the practice of empirically supported psychological interventions) of the American Psychological Association's Division of Clinical Psychology. Dr. Sanderson has published six books and more than 85 articles and chapters, primarily in the areas of anxiety, depression, personality disorders, and cognitive-behavioral therapy.

130111

Preface

Generalized anxiety disorder (GAD) is a prevalent and disabling clinical syndrome that requires treatment. Not only does it commonly occur on its own, but it is perhaps the most frequent comorbid diagnosis among patients with depressive disorders and other anxiety disorders as well. Thus clinicians are very likely to see many patients with GAD.

Only one psychosocial treatment—cognitive-behavioral therapy (CBT)—has a substantial body of empirical research supporting its efficacy with GAD. As a result, this treatment is an essential "tool" for any clinician treating adult outpatients.

This book was written to provide clinicians with a wide variety of empirically supported assessment and psychosocial treatment options. Within this framework, direction is given on how information from the assessment can be used to select and weave various treatment techniques into a comprehensive treatment plan for an individual patient. Each strategy is presented in extensive detail, so that the reader can implement these techniques on the basis of the descriptions provided. Detailed information is provided about treatment selection, rationale, and implementation. As much as possible, step-by-step instructions are provided. In order to bring the descriptions to life, case illustrations are included.

Although the effectiveness of the traditional CBT techniques outlined in this book is well established, these techniques are not without limitations. As is the case with many other empirically supported psychological and pharmacological treatments, many patients do not benefit. Recently there has been a proliferation of research on other techniques applied to GAD in efforts to improve treatment efficacy. Since these additional techniques are in the process of being subjected to well-controlled treatment outcome research, their efficacy has not yet been established. But ultimately they may prove useful with clients who do not respond well to traditional CBT alone. Though continued efforts need to be focused on improving this treatment, CBT is presently the best available psychotherapeutic intervention for GAD.

JAYNE L. RYGH and WILLIAM C. SANDERSON

Contents

List of Tables, Figures, and Handouts

TABLES

FIGURES

HANDOUTS

CHAPTER ONE

Generalized Anxiety Disorder
Diagnosis, Theories, and Treatment

DIAGNOSTIC CRITERIA

Generalized anxiety disorder (GAD) first appeared as a diagnostic category in the third edition of the *Diagnostic and Statistical Manual of Mental Disorders* (DSM-III; American Psychiatric Association [APA], 1980). But its clear definition as a disorder came only with significant revisions in the criteria for GAD made in DSM-III-R (APA, 1987). The last set of minor revisions of the criteria for GAD occurred in DSM-IV (APA, 1994). No further revisions were made in DSM-IV-TR (APA, 2000). The hallmark of GAD is now clearly defined by DSM-IV-TR as excessive and uncontrollable worry. Pathological worry is distinguished from nonpathological worry on the basis of the frequency, intensity, and duration of the worry; the individual's ability to control the worry; and whether the worry significantly interferes with functioning. In addition, nonpathological worry is less likely to be accompanied by the physiological symptoms that are present with pathological worry. Table 1.1 lists the DSM-IV-TR criteria for diagnosing GAD.

DIFFERENTIAL DIAGNOSIS

Various medical conditions and other organic factors can mimic symptoms of GAD. Underlying physical pathologies, such as disorders of the endocrine system (e.g., hyperthyroidism, pheochromocytoma, or hypercortisolism) or brain tumors, can present with symptoms similar to GAD. Other organic causes for an anxiety syndrome may include stimulant intoxication from caffeine, cocaine, or amphetamines; exposure to a toxin; or withdrawal from sedatives or alcohol.

1

TABLE 1.1. DSM-IV-TR Diagnostic Criteria for GAD

A. Excessive anxiety and worry (anxious expectation), occurring more days than not for at least 6 months, about a number of events or activities (such as work or school performance).

B. The person finds it difficult to control the worry.

C. The anxiety and worry are associated with three (or more) of the following six symptoms (with at least some symptoms present for more days than not for the past 6 months). **Note:** Only one item is required in children.

   (1) restlessness or feeling keyed up or on edge
   (2) being easily fatigued
   (3) difficulty concentrating or mind going blank
   (4) irritability
   (5) muscle tension
   (6) sleep disturbance (difficulty falling or staying asleep, or restless unsatisfying sleep)

D. The focus of the anxiety and worry is not confined to features of an Axis I disorder, e.g., the anxiety or worry is not about having a Panic Attack (as in Panic Disorder), being embarrassed in public (as in Social Phobia), being contaminated (as in Obsessive–Compulsive Disorder), being away from home or close relatives (as in Separation Anxiety Disorder), gaining weight (as in Anorexia Nervosa), having multiple physical complaints (as in Somatization Disorder), or having a serious illness (as in Hypochondriasis), and the anxiety and worry do not occur exclusively during Posttraumatic Stress Disorder.

E. The anxiety, worry, or physical symptoms cause clinically significant distress or impairment in social, occupational, or other important areas of functioning.

F. The disturbance is not due to the direct physiological effects of a substance (e.g., a drug of abuse, a medication) or a general medical condition (e.g., hyperthyroidism) and does not occur exclusively during a Mood Disorder, a Psychotic Disorder, or a Pervasive Developmental Disorder.

Note. From American Psychiatric Association (2000, p. 476). Copyright 2000 by the American Psychiatric Association. Reprinted by permission.

Anxiety and worry can be prominent features of many other psychiatric disorders, such as hypochondriasis, somatization disorder, eating disorders, and other anxiety disorders. In these instances, however, the themes of worry are clearly related to the other underlying disorders. Posttraumatic stress disorder, depressive disorders, and psychotic disorders also have general anxiety as a common feature. If the focus of anxiety and worry is exclusively related to one of these other disorders, a separate diagnosis of GAD would not be given.

When the symptoms occur within 3 months of the onset of a stressor and the stressor is present, a diagnosis of adjustment disorder with anxious mood would be given.

COEXISTING CONDITIONS

Research studies have indicated high rates of co-occurrence (ranging from 45% to 91%) of many other psychological disorders with GAD (Brawman-Mintzer & Lydiard, 1996). Certain medical conditions commonly coexist with GAD as well.

The Axis I diagnoses most frequently found to coexist with GAD include social phobia, panic disorder, specific phobia, major depressive disorder (MDD), and dysthymia (Brawman-Mintzer &

Lydiard, 1996; Brown & Barlow, 1992; Brown, Moras, Zinberg, & Barlow, 1993; Yonkers, Warshaw, Massion, & Keller, 1996). Other coexisting Axis I disorders include attention-deficit/hyperactivity disorder, trichotillomania, and stereotypic movement disorder (Stein, 2001). Individuals who have carried a diagnosis of GAD at some point in their lives also have high rates (42%) of MDD and dysthymic disorder (Sanderson, DiNardo, Rapee, & Barlow, 1990).

A recent study (Dyck et al., 2001) found a high coincidence (46%) of one or more Axis II disorders with GAD. Other studies have indicated rates ranging from 37% to 73%, with the most common coexisting personality disorders identified as avoidant, dependent, and mixed (Alnaes & Torgersen, 1999; Mavissakalian, Hamann, Haidaar, & DeGroot, 1995; Sanderson & Wetzler, 1991).

GAD has been found to be commonly associated with a variety of medical disorders. These disorders include chronic fatigue syndrome, irritable bowel syndrome, tension headaches, hypertension, diabetes, and heart disease (Stein, 2001).

PREVALENCE AND LIFE COURSE

The largest study to report prevalence data (using DSM-III-R criteria) indicates that rates of GAD are 1.6% and 5.8% for current and lifetime incidence, respectively (Wittchen, Zhao, Kessler, & Eaton, 1994). The highest risks are for adults 24 years and older; for those who have been previously married (separated, divorced, or widowed); and for homemakers. Other research has noted higher risks for blacks and females, with females outnumbering males by a ratio of 2.5:1 (Blazer, George, & Hughes, 1991). Individuals with GAD often report a long history dating back to childhood, with a large proportion unable to report a clear age of onset (Butler, Fennell, Robson, & Gelder, 1991; Noyes et al., 1992; Rapee, 1991; Sanderson & Barlow, 1990). One study (Carter, Wittchen, Pfister, & Kessler, 2001) found that the likelihood of being diagnosed with GAD increased significantly with age. Rapee (1991) has noted that if and when treatment is sought, it may be many years after a person becomes aware of symptoms. Treatment appears to be sought in most cases only after normal functioning has become grossly impaired by worry (Barlow, 2002). Spontaneous remission of the disorder is rare (Kessler et al., 1994). When remissions occur, relapse rates at 3 years have been substantial (27%), thus indicating a chronic relapsing course of the disorder (Yonkers, Dyck, Warshaw, & Keller, 2000). The chronicity of GAD and its resistance to treatment have led some researchers to conceptualize GAD more within the context of a personality disorder, although fluctuations in the disorder have been associated with recent life stressors and threatening events (Finlay-Jones & Brown, 1981; Blazer et al., 1991).

GENETIC FACTORS

One estimate indicates moderate heritability of 30% for GAD (Kendler, Neale, Kessler, Heath, & Eaves, 1992). Another estimate indicates modest heritability of about 15%–20%, with no gender-specific gene effects for GAD (Hettema, Prescott, & Kendler, 2001). However, most studies suggest a lack of specificity in the transmission of GAD (Weissman & Merikangas, 1986). By and large, the evidence suggests a more general heritability of traits, such as anxiety, negative affect, and behavioral inhibition in those with anxiety, depressive, and other related emotional disorders (Angst & Vollrath, 1991; Clark, Watson, & Mineka, 1994). Traits of neuroticism have been specifically positively correlated with anxiety and with anxiety disorders (Clark et al., 1994; Trull & Sher, 1994). Traits of high neuroticism and low extroversion have been found to indicate later vulnerability for anxiety and anxiety disorders (Gershuny & Sher, 1998). The general consensus is that there is a common genetic basis for anxiety and related disorders, such as depression, but that specific differences between disorders are best accounted for by environmental factors (e.g., Andrews, Stewart, Allen, & Henderson, 1990; Kendler et al., 1995).

ENVIRONMENTAL FACTORS

There is a dearth of studies on environmental factors related to GAD. In 1991, Rapee reviewed the existing research and noted that there were no prospective studies and only a few retrospective studies. He noted that of the existing studies, all compared subjects with panic disorder to subjects with GAD, and none of the studies included a control group of subjects without any clinically significant diagnoses for comparison. Since then, five studies have appeared in the literature.

Ben-Noun (1998) examined the relationship between persistent and prolonged family dysfunction and the rates of GAD in either parent. The results indicated that GAD developed in dysfunctional couples, and mostly within the female partners. Serious arguments, squabbles, and verbal or physical violence existed in these relationships. In addition, the presence of GAD in either partner appeared to produce a negative influence on the disturbed relationships within a family.

Barlow has hypothesized that overcontrolling family environments foster a diminished sense of personal control, leading to an external locus of control, which in turn contributes to increased negative affect and clinical symptoms of anxiety in children. This hypothesis is based on one aspect of Barlow's model of the nature and etiology of anxiety and its disorders, to be discussed later in this chapter (Barlow, 2002). Chorpita and Barlow (1998) evaluated this hypothesis through structural equation modeling and found a good fit with Barlow's model, lending preliminary support for the contribution of these factors to the development of GAD.

Lichtenstein and Cassidy (1991) found that individuals with GAD reported a higher incidence of enmeshed relationships and role reversals with primary caretakers, as well as more difficulty remembering their childhood. Borkovec (1994) found that subjects with GAD reported a higher incidence of past physical trauma in comparison with controls. Stober and Joorman (2001) found a relationship between amount of worry and parental criticism and expectations, but it is important to note that their subjects were college students rather than individuals diagnosed with GAD.

These studies suggest a possible role of dysfunction and/or trauma in the family environment for the development of GAD. However, much more research is required to clarify specific factors that might contribute to the development of this disorder.

Hudson and Rapee (2004) have presented a compelling preliminary etiological model of GAD. This model discusses potential interactive effects of genetics, individual temperament, parental anxiety, environmental support of avoidance, social-environmental influences, and external stressors in the development of the disorder. At present, this model is largely speculative, as it is mostly based on research on anxiety disorders in general rather than GAD specifically.

COSTS ASSOCIATED WITH GAD

GAD is one of the leading causes of workplace disability in the United States (Ballenger et al., 2001; Kessler, 2000). Sanderson and Andrews (2002) found that individuals in the general population who met DSM-IV criteria for GAD reported high levels of severe disability (42%). In another study using DSM-IV criteria (Wittcher, Carter, Pfister, Montgomery, & Kessler, 2000), GAD with and without coexisting MDD was associated with high levels of impairment in terms of reduction in activities and number of days completely lost. These findings are consistent with findings in other studies. Ormel et al. (1994) found that respondents with GAD reported a greater number of disability days, higher dysfunction in occupational roles, and high scores on reported physical disability. Kessler, DuPont, Bergllund, and Wittchen (1999) found that those with pure GAD reported significantly higher levels of social and work impairment and perceived their health as "only fair" or "poor," in comparison with respondents without GAD or MDD. The most impairment was found in those with comorbid GAD and MDD.

Additional costs associated with GAD are due to high rates of health care utilization (Ballenger et al., 2001; Greenberg et al., 1999). Approximately one-third of those with GAD seek medical attention for somatic symptoms (Bland, Newman & Orn, 1997). The medical specialists most often consulted are gastroenterologists (Kennedy & Schwab, 1997).

The chronic nature and high costs associated with GAD clearly indicate the necessity for effective treatments of this disabling disorder.

TREATMENT OUTCOME STUDIES

Treatments for GAD fall into two main categories: psychopharmacological and psychological. The following sections examine the outcome research on the treatments in each category.

Psychopharmacological Treatment

The majority of psychoactive medications prescribed for clients with GAD are benzodiazepines, azapirones (especially buspirone), tricyclic antidepressants (TCAs; e.g., imipramine), and selective serotonin–norepinephrine reuptake inhibitors (e.g., venlafaxine). Antipsychotic medications are also prescribed for GAD. The most commonly prescribed medications, with information regarding dosages and possible side effects, are listed in Table 1.2. Primary care physicians generally prescribe all of these medications.

The benzodiazepines tend to be frequently prescribed, as they provide immediate relief from anxiety. The side effects (e.g., fatigue that dissipates with continued use) are less noxious than those associated with most other classes of drugs. Abrupt withdrawal is associated with increased anxiety, sleep disturbances, agitation, headache, nausea, tremor, and (although rare) withdrawal

TABLE 1.2. Commonly Used Medications for Treating GAD

Brand (generic) name	Dosage (mg/day)	Common side effects
Benzodiazepines		
Ativan (lorazepam)	1–6	
Valium (diazepam)	5–40	
Xanax (alprazolam)	1–4	
Azapirones		Headache, nausea, dizziness, tension
BuSpar (buspirone)	20–40	
Antidepressants		
Selective serotonin–norepinephrine reuptake inhibitor		Nausea, somnolence, insomnia, sexual dysfunction, hypertension
Effexor (venlafaxine)	75–225	
Selective serotonin reuptake inhibitors (SSRIs)		Nausea, dyspepsia, diarrhea, insomnia, agitation, headache, decreased libido
Celexa (citalopram)	20–40	
Luvox (fluvoxamine)	100–200	
Paxil (paroxetine)	20–50	
Prozac (fluoxetine)	20–60	
Zoloft (sertraline)	50–200	
Tricyclic antidepressants (TCAs)		Dry mouth, constipation, urinary hesitance, orthostatic hypotension, hypertension, palpitations, tremor, sedation, stimulation, sexual dysfunction, weight gain
Adapin, Sinequan (doxepin)	150–300	
Elavil (amitriptyline)	150–300	
Norpramin (desipramine)	150–300	
Tofranil (imipramine)	150–300	

Note. This is not meant to be a complete list of medications. Only those commonly utilized benzodiazepines and TCAs are listed here. Based on Schatzberg, Cole, and DeBattista (1997) and Sussman and Stein (2001).

seizures. Over the last decade, however, evidence of problems with tolerance and dependence with long-term usage has led to increased concern and recommendations against using benzodiazepines as first-line agents in the pharmacotherapy of GAD (Rickels, DeMartinis, et al., 2000; Mahe & Balogh, 2000).

Buspirone (an azapirone) has gained popularity in the treatment of GAD because of reduced side effects. Buspirone is not sedating, does not interfere with psychomotor functioning, and has no withdrawal symptoms or abuse potential. Problems include reduced efficacy in patients with past usage of benzodiazepines, slower onset of action, and concerns about its potency with GAD (Ballenger, 1999). There is some evidence that it is more effective for patients with predominant psychic symptoms (worry, tension, and irritability) (Schweizer & Rickels, 1996).

Until recently, TCAs and selective serotonin reuptake inhibitors (SSRIs) were less commonly used. This was due to reduced compliance associated with anticholinergic side effects (e.g., constipation, urinary rention, weight gain, dry mouth, sexual dysfunction), delayed anxiolytic action, sedation, and orthostatic hypotension (primarily affecting elderly patients). Recent studies of a relatively new medication, venlafaxine (a combined serotonin–norepinephrine reuptake inhibitor) have indicated that it is better tolerated and effective for treatment of GAD without MDD

(Davidson, DuPont, Hedges, & Haskins, 1999; Rickels, Pollack, Sheehan, & Haskins, 2000; Meoni, Salinas, Brault, & Hackett, 2001). There are no serious withdrawal effects associated with this medication. As noted by Schatzberg, Cole, and DeBattista (1997), the SSRI antidepressants have not been shown to be more effective than earlier antidepressants such as TCAs. However, their more favorable side effect profile has resulted in SSRIs' frequently being selected as a first line of treatment over TCAs. Presently, venlafaxine extended release (XR) is the only antidepressant approved by the U.S. Food and Drug Administration for long-term management of GAD (Barman Balfour & Jarvis, 2000).

Antipsychotic medications (neuroleptics and major tranquilizers) are reported to be fairly commonly prescribed for GAD, despite textbook recommendations against doing so because of serious risks and a dearth of research on usage (El-Khayat & Baldwin, 1998). Short-term use of antipsychotics presents risks of sedation, acute dystonias, akathisia, and parkinsonism. Long-term use presents the risk of tardive dyskinesia, especially if treatment is interrupted.

Mahe and Balogh (2000) recently reviewed the literature on long-term treatment of GAD with psychoactive medications. As stated above, the most serious known problems with long-term usage are tolerance and dependence with the benzodiazepines. The authors concluded, however, that the results of their review were inconclusive, as adequate evaluations have not yet been performed.

Based on the research described above, we can make several recommendations:

1. Our most important recommendation is first to test the effectiveness of psychological intervention before introducing psychopharmacological treatment, except when the following conditions exist: when a client's functioning is significantly impaired by the disorder and an exclusive trial of psychological treatment creates undue hardship. When the level of anxiety is experienced as intolerable, medication as an adjunctive treatment may be necessary. But we also recommend the inclusion of a goal of becoming medication-free within treatment under such conditions. When the response to psychological intervention is present but has proved insufficient, we recommend that medication be considered as an adjunctive treatment.
2. Exclusive psychopharmacological treatment of GAD should be reserved for cases that prove to be highly refractory to psychological interventions.

These conservative recommendations are based on evidence of attenuated treatment gains upon withdrawal of medication; documented problems of tolerance and dependence associated with long-term usage of benzodiazepines; and lack of research on the risks associated with long-term psychopharmacological treatment of GAD.

Psychological Treatment

Many forms of psychological treatment have been applied to GAD, including psychoanalytic, brief supportive–expressive psychodynamic, supportive–expressive, and client-centered therapies; eye movement desensitization and reprocessing; electroencephalographic alpha and theta neurofeedback training; and cognitive-behavioral therapy (CBT). CBT, however, is the only form of psychological treatment for GAD that has been repeatedly subjected to rigorous, well-controlled treatment outcome research.

The various forms of CBT focus on symptom relief. More specifically, treatment is focused on relief of cognitive, somatic, and behavioral symptoms of GAD through the application of specified techniques. These techniques have included relaxation, systematic desensitization, applied relaxation (AR), cognitive restructuring (CR), worry exposure, stimulus control, response prevention, problem solving, pleasurable activity scheduling, interpersonal skills training, and assigned worry time.

Early studies comparing active forms of CBT with nondirective treatment or wait-list control conditions demonstrated greater improvement with active treatments than with no treatment (Barlow et al., 1984; Barlow, Rapee, & Brown, 1992; Blowers, Cobb, & Mathews, 1987; Butler, Cullington, Hibbert, Klimes, & Gelder, 1987; Lindsay, Gamsu, McLaughlin, Hood, & Espie, 1987). These studies typically involved cognitive therapy, relaxation training, anxiety management training, or some combination.

Many of the early studies comparing two or more active treatments, however, failed to show differential efficacy (Barlow et al., 1992; Blowers et al., 1987; Borkovec & Mathews, 1988; Durham & Turvey, 1987; Lindsay et al., 1987). These studies typically compared cognitive therapy with behavior therapy, CBT with nondirective therapy, or CBT with medication. The exceptions were studies by Borkovec et al. (1987) and Butler et al. (1991). Both of these studies indicated that the inclusion of a cognitive component produced superior results.

In a review of studies comparing CBT with nondirective therapy, Harvey and Rapee (1995) concluded that most studies clearly demonstrated that the inclusion of specific techniques, such as relaxation techniques and CR, led to marked reductions in the symptoms of GAD as compared with nondirective treatments. They suggested, however, that further research be conducted on the "nonspecific" effects within nondirective treatments, to determine exactly what produced the positive changes in GAD evidenced in these studies.

Well-controlled outcome studies that have utilized DSM-III-R and DSM-IV criteria include those by Butler et al. (1991), Barlow et al. (1992), White, Keenan, and Brooks (1992), Borkovec and Costello (1993), Durham et al. (1994), Öst and Breitholtz (2000), Ladouceur et al. (2000), and Borkovec, Newman, Pincus, and Lytle (2002). Only two of these studies compared CBT with a treatment from another orientation (Borkovec & Costello, 1993; Durham et al., 1994). All the other studies, with the exception of the Ladouceur et al. (2000) study, compared differing combinations of cognitive therapy, CBT, behavior therapy, and/or AR. The Ladouceur et al. (2000) study found significant improvement (77%) with a version of CBT that targeted intolerance of uncertainty, erroneous beliefs about worry, poor problem orientation, and cognitive avoidance in comparison with a delayed-treatment condition.

Borkovec and Costello (1993) compared AR, CBT, and nondirective therapy. AR and CBT were equivalent and superior to nondirective therapy at posttreatment. At the 12-month follow-up, CBT was found to be superior to AR. In a later study conducted by Öst and Breitholtz (2000), however, both AR and cognitive therapy produced similar results at posttreatment and a 1-year follow-up. In this study, both conditions produced clinically significant improvement in approximately two-thirds of the subjects in both groups. These results were similar to those in a study by Borkovec et al. (2002), which compared AR and self-control desensitization (S-CD), cognitive therapy, and a combination of these methods. Significant improvements in anxiety and depression were maintained for 2 years. No differences were found between the conditions. However, these researchers found that interpersonal problems were negatively associated with posttherapy and follow-up improvements.

Durham et al. (1994) compared cognitive therapy, analytic psychotherapy, and anxiety management training under high- and low-intensity contact conditions. High-intensity contact consisted of 16–20 sessions lasting 1 hour each over 6 months. Low-intensity contact consisted of 8–10 sessions of the same length over the same period. The results indicated that cognitive therapy was significantly more effective than analytic psychotherapy. At a 6-month follow-up, the superiority of cognitive therapy was even greater, as treatment gains were maintained in the cognitive therapy group. Anxiety management produced results similar to those of cognitive therapy, but the most durable and broad-based improvements occurred with cognitive therapy at posttreatment and follow-up. A 1-year follow-up of this study (Durham et al., 1999) indicated that differences between the low-intensity contact conditions were less evident. The most positive outcomes occurred in the high-intensity cognitive therapy condition, with approximately two-thirds maintaining clinically significant improvement.

Borkovec and Ruscio (2001) reviewed outcomes of 13 controlled clinical trials that included CBT, cognitive therapy, behavior therapy, placebo or nonspecific treatment, and psychodynamic treatment of GAD. They concluded that CBT produced the most intermediate and long-term improvement in both anxiety and depression as compared to no treatment, nonspecific treatment, and psychodynamic treatment. CBT occasionally produced greater effects than either cognitive or behavior therapy alone.

Fisher and Durham (1999) reviewed the studies that used DSM-III-R and DSM-IV criteria. They concluded that CBT and AR produced the highest overall recovery rates. Approximately 60% showed significant improvement and 40% recovered from the disorder, as evidenced at 6-month follow-ups to these types of treatment. Other types of treatment showed much more modest recovery rates (30% or less). These rates are similar to the 50% high-end-state improvement rates of GAD noted in other reviews (Borkovec & Whisman, 1996; Chambless & Gillis, 1993).

Gould, Otto, Pollack, and Yap (1997) conducted a meta-analysis of controlled studies utilizing CBT and/or pharmacotherapy with GAD. No statistical differences were found between the two forms of treatment, with both clearly efficacious at posttreatment. Only CBT, however, produced significantly greater effects on the severity of coexisting depression at posttreatment. Moreover, the long-term effects indicated that treatment gains were maintained with CBT, whereas gains were attenuated following medication discontinuation.

Studies on long-term maintenance (6 months or more after treatment) of treatment gains indicate that the gains with various cognitive and/or behavior therapies and AR are maintained (Barlow et al., 1992; Borkovec & Costello, 1993; Borkovec & Mathews, 1988; Butler et al., 1987, 1991; Durham et al., 1999; White, 1998). In addition, long-term outcome data in several studies indicate substantial reductions in usage of anxiolytic medications with these treatments (Barlow et al., 1992; Butler et al., 1991; Durham et al., 1999; White et al., 1992). This is notable, given that benzodiazepines are particularly refractory to discontinuation (Rickels, De Martinis, et al., 2000; Schweizer & Rickels, 1996, 1997).

Newman (2000) suggested numerous factors that potentially contribute to nonresponse to CBT of GAD. These factors include interpersonal difficulties, personality disorders, severity of symptoms, Axis I comorbidity, low motivation for treatment, and avoidance of emotion. Relatively few studies of these factors as they are specifically related to GAD exist at this time. Two studies of note are those by Sanderson, Beck, and McGinn (1994) and Durham, Allan, and Hackett (1997). Sanderson et al. (1994) found no effect of Axis II disorders on treatment outcome. Durham et al. (1997) used logistic regression to investigate the validity of various predictors on improvement and relapse following treatment. They found the best predictor of sustained improvement to be significant relationship status, type of treatment, and socioeconomic status. Marriage or cohabitation increased odds of a favorable outcome; the quality of the relationship moderated this factor, however. CBT also increased the odds of a favorable outcome, as did higher socioeconomic status and a primary diagnosis of GAD without comorbid Axis I diagnoses. A positive therapeutic relationship also made a small but significant contribution to improvement. History of past treatment reduced the probability of improvement. Predictors of relapse included being single, widowed, or divorced; receiving analytic therapy (instead of cognitive therapy in this study); Axis I comorbidity; and a withdrawn, isolated, schizoid lifestyle.

Durham et al.'s (1997) results are similar to those factors found to be predictive of poor prognosis of GAD in other studies (Angst & Vollrath, 1991; Mancuso, Townsend, & Mercante, 1993; Yonkers et al., 2000). These other studies, however, did not focus on prognostic factors specific to CBT. Although Durham et al.'s results may provide helpful information regarding potential poor response or nonresponse to CBT, it is important that these results be viewed with caution, as they have not yet been cross-validated.

The research described above indicates that the most positive short- and long-term outcomes have been obtained with CBT and/or relaxation techniques. Although the specific techniques for either type of treatment have not been held constant across all studies, the general principles and practices have been consistent. Later chapters of this book present the general principles and practices of CBT and relaxation techniques, as well as the specific variations of the techniques utilized in the above-described studies. However, it is important to reiterate that a large percentage (approximately 30%–40%) of those with GAD do not significantly benefit from the most effective treatments. This is in contrast to the higher clinical improvement rates found with CBT of other anxiety disorders (e.g., panic disorder, with nonresponder rates between 20% and 25%). The prevalence and costs of GAD are significant incentives for improving these response rates. In an effort to speed this goal, we present information on additional techniques new to a CBT context that has shown potential promise. These techniques include those that target interpersonal problems and emotional avoidance. Both are factors hypothesized by Newman (2000) to contribute to nonresponse to traditional CBT for GAD. Most of these techniques are presented in Chapter 8, with a few in Chapters 5 and 6. Those techniques that have not yet received strong empirical support are identified as such when presented in this book. The application of any technique requires careful assessment to determine effectiveness. Expertise and flexibility in the application of a wide variety of effective techniques, in addition to a willingness to experiment with newly developed techniques, may enhance positive treatment outcomes. Clearly, more research is needed for a more complete base of knowledge about GAD and its treatment.

BEHAVIORAL AND COGNITIVE THEORIES OF ANXIETY DISORDERS, AND RELATED TREATMENT TECHNIQUES

Many of the CBT techniques that have been found effective in the treatment outcome research are presented throughout this book. Understanding their effective use, however, requires knowledge of the behavioral and cognitive theories behind these techniques. We review these theories here.

Behavioral Theory

Behavioral theories of anxiety disorders and the techniques drawn from them are based on the principles of classical and operant conditioning. In particular, Mowrer's (1947) two-factor theory of fear, which relies on the interplay of classical and operant conditioning, underlies some of the most effective techniques for anxiety reduction to date.

Classical conditioning explains how an anxiety response to nonthreatening stimuli can develop. It is a process of learning by association. When something that is already feared is paired with something that is otherwise neutral, the person learns to fear what was previously neutral.

Operant conditioning principles explain how fear or anxiety responses can be maintained or increased. Responses are increased or decreased through reward or punishment, respectively. Negative reinforcement is a special case of operant conditioning where punishment is either terminated or avoided with a response. Such responses are rewarded by the nonoccurrence of punishment. The well-known "fight" and "flight" responses are examples of responses that can be maintained or increased through this process.

Mowrer's two-factor theory explains the development and maintenance of fear or anxiety through classical conditioning and negative reinforcement. An example is a person's development of an anxiety response to elevators as the result of having been trapped in one. Following this experience, the person consistently avoids elevators. By doing so, the person effectively prevents further experiences of punishment in elevators. The conditioned fear of elevators and the behavioral response of avoiding elevators are maintained through this process.

These principles have been extended to cognitive (Borkovec, 1979) and to internal physiological (Barlow, 2002) responses. Theories that have incorporated these extensions are presented in later sections.

Behavioral techniques for anxiety reduction based upon the theory described above include systematic desensitization, exposure, scheduled worry time, and response prevention. Systematic desensitization (Wolpe, 1958) is a form of counterconditioning. It works to break down the association between a stimulus and the fear response. The procedure consists of countering a conditioned anxiety response (e.g., physiological arousal) with a deep relaxation response during imaginal presentations of a feared stimulus. A new conditioned response, relaxation, is learned to replace the old one of fear and physical tension. Exposure is based on the concept of extinction, which is another way to break down conditioned associations. Scheduled worry time reduces the development of new fear triggers through conditioned association and weakens existing associations. Response prevention is a behavioral technique that prevents habitual flight and fight responses. Specific behaviors addressed with this technique are escape, avoidance, procrastination, overpreparation, checking, and reassurance seeking. It allows clients to learn they are still safe without either flight or fight responses. Multiple variations and extensions of these techniques exist for anxiety reduction (e.g., S-CD, AR, stimulus control, imaginal exposure, *in vivo* exposure).

Cognitive Theory

The most influential cognitive theorist on anxiety disorders is Beck (see especially Beck & Emery with Greenberg, 1985). Beck emphasizes the cognitive factors that are operating in cases where emotions, such as anxiety, are inappropriate or exaggerated. He believes that inaccurate perceptions of danger are responsible for the activation, control, and modulation of emotional behavior responses associated with anxiety disorders. Beck states that overactive cognitive schemas about danger underlie these perceptions. According to Beck, individuals with anxiety disorders process information about internal and external events through heightened activity of these schemas. When such schemas are activated, events are more likely to be perceived as threatening to vital interests. Conceptualizations and cognitive processing of experiences become highly selective. Dysfunctional thinking processes, such as catastrophizing, selective abstraction, and dichotomous thinking, become evident and magnify the sense of danger or vulnerability.

Beck suggests that much of this processing occurs outside of conscious awareness. Consequently, the activation of anxiety can be contrary to conscious intent and independent of controlled, rational thought processes.

Beck has introduced the notion that inappropriate and exaggerated anxiety can be reduced through rational confrontation of distorted thinking and of danger schemas with a Socratic method of questioning. Cognitive techniques have been developed to help clients monitor and restructure their cognitions. In addition, behavioral experimentation has been included as an aid to restructuring cognitions.

Cognitive-Behavioral Theories

Lang's Model

Lang's model of anxiety disorders (Lang, 1978, 1979, 1985, 1994; Lang, Cuthbert, & Bradley, 1998) presumes the existence of an emotion memory structure consisting of three categories of information stored in the form of stimulus, response, and meaning propositions. Lang presumes that this emotion memory structure is stored in long-term memory and can be activated by or processed in short-term memory when external and/or internal cues tap the associated propositions of the structure. As such, various stimuli, responses, or interpretations of stimuli or responses can evoke this structure and produce the various cognitive, behavioral, and physiological aspects of emotional responding.

Lang proposes that the degree of associative coherence in the affective memory network differs with each of the anxiety disorders. Lang places the disorders on a continuum from tight to fluid as follows: focal phobia; obsessions and compulsions; social anxiety; agoraphobia; panic; and generalized anxiety states. Focal phobias and obsessions and compulsion are considered the most tightly coherent; generalized anxiety is considered a condition with the maximum associative fluidity of affective response structures. The degree of associative fluidity determines the extent to which these response dispositions "float" in memory and can be activated by specific stimuli. The more fluid the associations, the more that different stimuli can evoke an emotional response. The effectiveness of CBT techniques is presumably related to how well this emotion memory structure is activated throughout the course of treatment.

Barlow's Theory

Barlow (2002) has developed a theory of anxiety disorders that further elaborates the model presented by Lang. Based on clinical and phenomenological evidence, Barlow (2002) posits that generalized anxiety (or anxious apprehension) and panic (or fear) are two distinct, broad-based phenomena present in all anxiety disorders to varying degrees. Barlow's emotion theory of anxiety disorders highlights generalized anxiety (or anxious apprehension) as the major feature of all anxiety disorders.

Anxious apprehension is primarily characterized by a sense of an inability to predict or control future events that are personally salient. It is described as a state of high negative affect that is part of a diffuse cognitive–affective structure. Chronic tendencies of sensing events as unpredictable and/or uncontrollable presumably result from a developmental history in which opportunities to predict or control both aversive (e.g., punishment) and appetitive (e.g., attention, food, etc.) stimuli were insufficient. Parenting styles of noncontingent and/or negatively contingent (via overprotective, intrusive, or punitive) responses to a child's attempts to control vital events in the environment presumably produced a cognitive template of an external locus of control within the child. Barlow considers an external locus of control a major psychological vulnerability factor for the development of anxiety disorders. Barlow posits that anxious apprehension is a state of helplessness caused by the perception that one is unable to predict, control, or obtain vital results, with a strong physiological substrate of arousal or readiness for counteracting this state of helplessness.

In contrast, panic is described as a coherent emotional response possibly "hard-wired" to danger that is present or imminent. Barlow suggests that the threshold for panic is very likely to be genetically determined, due to the survival value of this response. Panic may occur predictably in situations where well-being is threatened (e.g., falling off a cliff, being bitten by a snake, etc.), or unpredictably in situations where there are no clearly observable antecedents for this response. The former instances of panic are termed "true alarms" and the latter "false alarms." Panic also may occur as the result of learning. "Learned alarms" develop when this fear response becomes conditioned to various internal and/or external stimuli.

According to Barlow, an anxiety disorder can be said to exist only if there is anxious apprehension over the possibility of experiencing an alarm response or any other type of negative event in the future. The negative affect associated with the sense of unpredictability and/or uncontrollability can be evoked by a variety of external and internal cues. Once evoked, anxious apprehension is a response that relies heavily on various cognitive processes. The cues that evoke anxious apprehension presumably tap the cognitive–affective structure of associated stimulus, response, and/or meaning propositions stored in long-term memory theorized by Lang.

The process of anxious apprehension involves a vicious feedback cycle. This cycle begins once this diffuse cognitive–affective structure is evoked. In essence, the sense of unpredictability and/or uncontrollability, and the accompanying physiological arousal, compel the individual's attention inward. This shift to self-evaluative concerns increases arousal further. Increased arousal causes attention to narrow. The individual begins to focus even more closely on the unpleasant affect and on his or her sense that future events are unpredictable and/or uncontrollable. This encourages further processing of self-evaluative content, leading to further increases in arousal, and so on. Ultimately, attention becomes so narrowed that performance and concentration are disrupted. Attempts to cope include avoidance of specific cues evocative of this state, as well as worrying. Worrying is a coping strategy that quells negative affect through (often futile) efforts to plan and solve problems.

THEORIES OF GAD

Three theories specific to GAD—one developed by Wells, another by Ladouceur and colleagues, and the third by Borkovec—have been formulated on the basis of empirical evidence related to excessive and uncontrollable worry in GAD. Although all three theories are based on recent evidence regarding worry, the fit of each model exclusively to GAD has not yet been fully evaluated and determined.

Wells's Metacognitive Theory

Wells (1995, 1999) has presented a metacognitive theory of GAD that accounts for the development and maintenance of excessive and uncontrollable worry. "Metacognition" refers to knowledge, beliefs, and appraisals about cognition, as well as regulation and awareness of ongoing cognition. This model describes GAD as the result of "interaction between the motivated use of worry as a coping strategy, negative appraisal of worry, and worry control attempts" (1995, p. 301). The model separates worry into two types. Type 1 refers to worry about external events and noncognitive internal events, such as bodily sensations. The events associated with Type 1 worry may be real or imagined events. Worry associated with specific phobias (e.g., fear of heights) or panic disorder may primarily involve Type 1 worry. Type 2 refers to worry about one's own thinking or worry about worry (termed "metaworry"). Wells proposes that the key feature of GAD is metaworry.

Wells posits that individuals with GAD hold both positive negative beliefs about worry. Positive beliefs are that worry serves a protective or coping function—for example, that it prevents, contains, or helps one avoid negative events. Negative beliefs are that Type 1 worry is maladaptive or harmful—for example, it interferes with effective and efficient on-task functioning, and/or has deleterious effects on one's physical and/or psychological health. Because both positive and negative beliefs about Type 1 worry are held simultaneously, individuals with GAD are described as being in a state of metacognitive dissonance or conflict about worry. As noted above, metaworry (Type 2 worry) occurs when the individual begins to worry about worrying. Attempts to suppress worry, however, only serve to increase the intrusiveness of worry.

According to Well's model, problematic worry develops over time. It begins with a tendency to use worry as a coping strategy for real or imagined threats. This strategy may develop through modeling, in which parents advocated worry as a positive coping strategy, or through experiences where worry was followed by nonoccurrences of aversive events, leading to beliefs in the protective powers of worry. Metaworry eventually develops as a result of various pathways. One pathway is that as worry becomes increasingly automated through overuse, it becomes increasingly disruptive and stimulates attempts to control the worry. However, because attempts to suppress worry only increase its intrusiveness, beliefs begin to be formulated regarding this decrease in control over one's mental activities. A second pathway occurs as the result of positive beliefs about worry or beliefs that worry is uncontrollable. These beliefs decrease efforts to manage worry, thereby augmenting the intrusiveness of worry. As a consequence, beliefs about impairments in one's ability to control the worry may develop or be strengthened. Third, observed negative life events associated with worry in others may lead to beliefs that worry is harmful or dangerous. Fourth, blocking of emotional processing via worry increases intrusions and decreases perceptions of mental control.

Behavioral strategies of avoidance maintain both types of worry. Behavioral avoidance of feared situations is associated with Type 1 worry. Behavioral avoidance of situations that trigger worry, reassurance seeking, checking, and behavioral self-control is associated with Type 2 worry. The avoidance strategies for Type 1 worry preserve positive beliefs about worry, whereas such strategies for Type 2 worry preserve negative beliefs associated with worry. Nonoccurrences of catastrophe following avoidance motivated by either type of worry maintain both positive and negative beliefs about worry.

Wells (1995) recommends a treatment focus on challenging metaworry, with the aim of developing more adaptive metacognitive knowledge. To facilitate acquisition of new knowledge, clients should be taught to "let go" of worries, as opposed to pursuing active strategies to control worry. Positive and negative metabeliefs about worry should be restructured. If worry is highly automatic, clients should learn to use disengagement strategies as soon as worry is recognized; however, it is important that the clients not use this as a control strategy to avoid specific fears (such as insanity) regarding worry.

The Four-Part Model of Ladouceur and Colleagues

Ladouceur and colleagues (Ladouceur, Blais, Freeston, & Dugas, 1998; Ladouceur, Talbot, & Dugas, 1997) have presented a model for the acquisition and maintenance of GAD that identifies four main variables: intolerance of uncertainty, beliefs about worry, poor problem orientation, and cognitive avoidance.

The first and most important variable in this model is intolerance of uncertainty. This intolerance is the result of lowered thresholds for ambiguity, stronger reactions to ambiguity, and anticipation of threatening outcomes as a consequence of uncertainty. Intolerance of uncertainty leads to dysfunctional behaviors (such as seeking excessive amounts of evidence to increase certainty) that interfere with effective problem solving.

The second feature of this model consists of beliefs about worry. Individuals with GAD tend to overestimate the advantages and to underestimate the disadvantages of worry. Worry is believed to serve helpful and protective purposes (e.g., to prevent bad things from happening). The nonoccurrence of feared events following worry confirms these beliefs.

The third feature is poor problem orientation. Problem orientation is a higher-order meta-cognitive activity; it is not a specific set of problem-solving skills. More specifically, poor problem orientation consists of poor problem-solving confidence and poor perceived control over the problem-solving process.

The fourth feature is cognitive avoidance of threatening mental images. This feature is based on Borkovec's avoidance theory of worry, which is presented in more detail in the next section.

Dugas, Gagnon, Ladouceur, and Freeston (1998) suggest that clinical treatment of GAD should focus primarily on increasing tolerance of uncertainty by challenging assumptions that uncertainty can and should be avoided. In addition, beliefs about worry should be reevaluated with CR techniques. These authors suggest a differentiation of worry based on whether it is about immediate problems or about improbable events in the future. Treatment of worry on immediate problems should target intolerance of uncertainty and poor problem orientation. Poor problem orientation can be addressed by teaching the client to stay focused on the key elements of the problem situation and to ignore associated minor details. Once key elements of the problem are identified, problem solving is to proceed on those key elements, despite uncertainties regarding outcome. In essence, the treatment teaches the client to reach a compromise between avoiding the problem and gathering excessive information to eliminate uncertainty. Treatment of worry about improbable events in the future will require cognitive exposure to threatening images, while using covert response prevention.

Borkovec's Avoidance Theory

Borkovec (see especially Borkovec, Alcaine, & Behar, 2004) has presented an avoidance theory of worry for GAD. In 1990, research conducted by Borkovec and Inz established that the nature of the worry is predominantly thought rather than imaginal activity. This finding led Borkovec and Inz to speculate that the predominance of thought in worry may serve as a motivated form of cognitive avoidance of affective imagery. This idea was based on Lang's (1985) notion that somatic activation of emotion occurs by way of imagery. Borkovec suggests that worry is a highly motivated process in which somatic activity evoked by affective imagery is avoided or dampened with excessive conceptual activity. He theorizes that the chronic and difficult-to-control worry found in GAD is motivated not only by the need to find a solution to a problem (a perceived threat), but also by its ability to suppress somatic activity. The negative reinforcement from the nonoccurrence or termination of negative external and internal events strengthens this cognitive avoidance response. Based on recent research, Borkovec theorizes that the superficial content of worry may serve additionally as a means of avoiding more emotionally distressing topics (possibly related to past trauma, early negative attachment experiences, or current interpersonal problems).

Borkovec's treatment for GAD consists of the following elements:

1. *Response prevention.* Clients are taught to establish "worry periods" and/or "worry-free zones." Worry periods are selected times and places where worry is permitted each day. Worry-free zones are times when worry, if detected, is postponed until the individual is out of those

zones. Over time, the worry-free zones are expanded to include more places, times, and activities. Both of these techniques are discussed in Chapter 5.

2. *Worry outcome monitoring.* Clients are instructed to record worries with associated feared outcomes, as well as the actual outcomes on a daily basis. Worry outcome monitoring increases awareness that perceptions of future threat are overestimated and coping abilities underestimated. Techniques for increasing this awareness are presented in Chapters 3 and 5.

3. *Present-moment focus of attention.* Multiple methods of relaxation (progressive muscular relaxation [PMR], meditation, diaphragmatic breathing [DB], and relaxing imagery) and CR techniques are taught to help the client both live more fully in the present moment and experiment with multiple ways of being. These techniques are presented in Chapters 5, 6, and 8.

4. *Imagery.* S-CD (presented in Chapter 6), followed by imagining effective coping and the most likely realistic outcomes, is used to create a new alternate set of historical records stored in memory through imagination.

5. *Targeting core fears avoided through worry.* Borkovec suggests that earlier trauma, attachment difficulties, and/or current interpersonal difficulties may be related to emotional distress from unmet needs in the client's life. Techniques that address these issues are currently being explored by Newman, Castonguay, Borkovec, and Molnar (2004). These techniques are presented in Chapter 8.

CONCLUSIONS

The research clearly indicates that CBT for GAD is effective and generally produces the most positive long-term results. This book provides detailed information about the most effective CBT techniques and their implementation. In addition, this book presents information about newly developed techniques with potential promise. Chapter 2 reviews the available techniques and provides a general summary of the empirical support for various techniques.

CHAPTER TWO

A General Description of Treatment

OVERVIEW OF THE MODEL USED IN TREATMENT

In Chapter 1, we have discussed the main theoretical ideas of Mowrer (classical and operant conditioning of fear responses), Beck (cognitive appraisal), Lang (the associative network), Barlow (uncontrollability), Wells (metaworry), Ladouceur and colleagues (intolerance of uncertainty and poor problem orientation), and Borkovec (worry as cognitive avoidance of emotional experience). These theories can be subsumed within a relatively simple model that can be used in treatment. To facilitate both clinicians' and clients' understanding of GAD, we divide the experience of anxiety into three different parts: the cognitive, the physiological, and the behavioral. A fourth component is included in the model to account for stimuli that trigger episodes of worry. (Figure 2.1 provides a visual representation of the model; Table 2.1 offers examples of the model's four components.)

We make a distinction between adaptive and nonadaptive anxiety. Anxiety is neither good nor bad. It is simply an emotion that can serve either adaptive or nonadaptive functions. The goal of treatment is not to eliminate anxiety; rather, it is to maintain adaptive forms of anxiety and markedly reduce those that are nonadaptive. In other words, the main goal for treating GAD is to reduce episodes of nonadaptive anxiety and worry.

During episodes of anxiety and worry, there is a perception of potential threat to vital interests, and preparatory or avoidant responses to that threat occur. The perception of and responses to threat are apparent in specific cognitive, physiological, and behavioral activities.

Anxiety and worry are adaptive when they assist in the accurate identification of potential threat and motivates appropriate coping responses to threat. Nonadaptive anxiety and worry occur when potential threat is inaccurately assessed and/or when inappropriate coping responses are activated. Presumably, inaccurate perceptions and problematic coping responses develop and

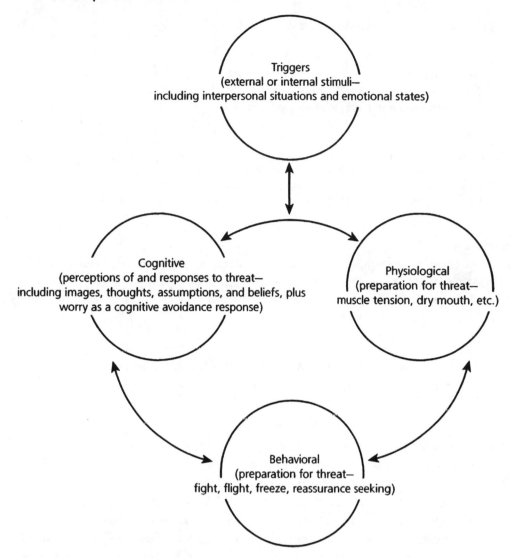

FIGURE 2.1. The experience of anxiety and worry.

are maintained through a variety of classical and operant conditioning experiences over time. In those with GAD, excessive numbers and degrees of stimuli (both external and internal) have become classically conditioned to trigger fear. In addition, ineffective coping responses to fear have developed and have been maintained through the process of negative reinforcement. These excessive conditioned associations are evident in the cognitive, physiological, and behavioral symptoms of GAD. The treatment techniques in this book focus on altering the cognitive, physiological, and behavioral symptoms of GAD by weakening various conditioned associations. We now describe each part of the model in more detail.

The cognitive component of GAD in this model consists of perceptions of threat, as well as cognitive responses to these threat perceptions. Cognitive activity is apparent in images, thoughts, assumptions, and/or beliefs. Perceptions of danger or threat to vital interests may be re-

TABLE 2.1. The Components of the Anxiety Experience, with Examples

Cognitive components

Perceptions: Beliefs, assumptions, thoughts, and/or images about danger, vulnerability, threats to vital interests, and/or threats to one's coping resources.

Responses: Excess cognitive planning, preparation, and/or avoidance.

Physiological component

Physiological mobilization: Muscle tension, restlessness, trembling, twitching, shaking, shallow breathing, heart palpitations and/or tachycardia, dry mouth, difficulty swallowing, cold and/or clammy hands, sweating, hot flashes or chills, frequent urination, aches, soreness, nausea, diarrhea, or constipation. Also, increased sympathetic nervous system activity and reduced flexibility in parasympathetic nervous system.

Behavioral component

Flight behaviors: Avoidance, procrastination, evasion, escape, and reassurance seeking (requests for support, advice, and/or assistance).

Fight behaviors: Checking, overprotection, and reassurance seeking.

Freeze behaviors: Stammered speech and halted behavior.

Triggers

External stimuli: Any stimuli conditioned with fear, including interpersonal situations.

Internal stimuli: Mental images, physiological sensations, emotional states.

sponses to specific stimuli (internal or external). For example, a sense of danger could be triggered by an internal image of one's child being hit by a car while bicycling on neighborhood streets. A lightning storm could be interpreted as putting one's life and home in grave danger. Images, thoughts, assumptions, and/or beliefs may convey a general vulnerability to negative outcomes ("Things never go right for me") or an inability to predict or control events (internal, environmental, or social) as they relate to the self. Cognitions may also function as coping responses to specific threat-associated stimuli (internal or external). For example, an individual may engage in excess planning for a minor threat as a way to avoid emotional distress from a much more serious threat (e.g., a woman worries excessively about minor matters to avoid facing severe marital problems). Cognitions may be related to the individual's sense of personal adequacy or inadequacy to cope with threat. For example, an individual may believe that his or her problem-solving abilities provide insufficient protection against harm. The cognitions may contain both positive and negative beliefs about worry and the problem-solving process. For example, an individual may believe that worry helps to prevent catastrophe, but also may believe that worry will damage his or her health.

The physiological component of GAD consists of innate physiological responses that support instinctive action under conditions of danger or threat. The sensations associated with this physiological mobilization may include muscle tension, restlessness, trembling, twitching, shaking, shallow breathing, heart palpitations and/or tachycardia, dry mouth, difficulty swallowing, cold and/or clammy hands, sweating, hot flashes or chills, and frequent urination. When physiological mobilization is prolonged or frequent, as in GAD, additional sensations of aches or soreness, nausea, and diarrhea or constipation may be noticed. The excessive physiological mobilization in GAD is evidenced in increased activity in the sympathetic division and reduced flexibility in the parasympathetic division of the autonomic nervous system.

As do fear responses to perceived imminent threat, the behavioral component of GAD in this model appears as both flight and fight behaviors. Flight behaviors include avoidance, evasion, escape, and procrastination. Overpreparation, checking, and overprotection are examples of fight behaviors. Reassurance seeking may be either a flight or a fight behavior: It is flight when the purpose is to flee to a protective figure, but it is fight when the purpose is excessive checking. It appears as repeated requests for support, advice, or assistance.

When one component of GAD in this model is activated, other components can be automatically activated by way of association. As such, this model does not necessarily depend upon cognitive appraisals for the elicitation and/or maintenance of GAD. An example is as follows. A woman is lying in her bed. The backfire from a car activates an innate startle response. The physical arousal propels a state of hypervigilance. The woman notices other sounds inside the house. An image of a burglar breaking into the house pops into her mind. She tries to suppress the image, but another image of an intruder in her daughter's bedroom surfaces. She notices the pounding of her heart. Her breath is shallow and quick. She thinks about calling the police, but lies still for fear of making any noise. She thinks of taking a letter opener with her while planning to inspect the house. Another image surfaces of being strangled by the intruder. Her chest is tight, and her breath is rapid. She carefully and quietly gets out of bed, taking the letter opener with her, and begins to look around. She checks the hallway, then her children in their bedrooms, and then the bathroom. She hesitates at the top of the stairway. Feeling tense while intent on listening, she thinks that the intruder may have heard her movements and is lying low. She stands there waiting, watching, and listening. Eventually, after several minutes of seeing nothing unusual and hearing no new sounds, she returns to her bed. Her high state of arousal makes her unable to sleep, however. Other worrisome scenarios come to mind over the next sleepless hour. In this case, physical arousal triggers the worry by evoking images of danger that keep the arousal going.

The techniques presented within this book teach clients to recognize and alter erroneous images of danger, physiological mobilization, and problematic responses, as well as problematic appraisals of stimuli of the worry process. Many different techniques are used for these purposes, and these are reviewed next. For ease of discussion, the techniques for treating GAD are grouped according to specific targets. It is important to note, however, that each technique has the potential for indirectly affecting other targets. Table 2.2 lists the techniques presented in this book. The following sections provide brief descriptions of the techniques; following these descriptions, empirical support for these techniques is reviewed briefly. Chapters 5 through 8 provide extensive descriptions of each group of techniques, with examples of implementation.

TECHNIQUES THAT TARGET THE COGNITIVE COMPONENT

The cognitive component of GAD can be modulated with a wide variety of techniques. These techniques include psychoeducation, cognitive restructuring (CR), hypothesis testing, positive imagery, worry exposure, improving problem orientation, cost–benefit analysis of coping, and two cognitive response prevention techniques: scheduled worry time and worry-free zones.

TABLE 2.2. Overview of Techniques That Target Components of GAD

Target: Cognitive component	Target: Physiological component	Target: Behavioral component	Target: Associated problems
Psychoeducation	Progressive muscular relaxation (PMR)	Behavioral response prevention	Mindfulness (for experiential avoidance)
Cognitive restructuring (CR)	Diaphragmatic breathing (DB)	*In vivo* exposure	Emotional processing and regulation training (for emotion regulation without worry)
Worry Episode Log (for Treatment)	Self-control desensitization (S-CD)	Pleasurable activity scheduling	
Guided discovery	Applied relaxation (AR)		Interpersonal effectiveness (for unmet needs)
Decatastrophizing			Time management (to let go of unnecessary worry-induced behaviors)
Developing alternative viewpoints			
Hypothesis testing			
Positive imagery			
Worry exposure			
Improving problem orientation			
Cost–benefit analysis of coping			
Cognitive response prevention			
Scheduled worry time			
Worry-Free Zones			

The first technique, psychoeducation, is the provision of corrective information through direct education. This is aimed at altering any misconception about the nature and function of fear, anxiety, and worry. This education is provided through didactic means in session and is crucial to socializing the client to treatment (see Chapter 4).

The CR technique is based upon Beck's model (see Beck & Emery with Greenberg, 1985). This technique provides the client with a tool for critically evaluating and modifying his or her interpretations of and responses to environmental or internal stimulus events.

CR is accomplished in four basic steps. First, images, thoughts, assumptions, and beliefs associated with episodes of worry are brought into full awareness through several methods. These methods include self-monitoring with the treatment version of the Worry Episode Log (see Handout 5.1 in Chapter 5), juxtaposing facts and interpretations of facts, identifying common cognitive distortions, and uncovering core beliefs. Second, cognitions are systematically confronted and evaluated with the methods of guided discovery and decatastrophizing. Guided discovery utilizes a Socratic method to question the validity of cognitions. Decatastrophizing is used to confront avoidance of emotionally distressing cognitions, so that more realistic appraisals become possible. Third, the client is assisted in developing alternative viewpoints with such methods as taking a third-person perspective, switching roles, changing the frame, and others. Fourth, clients are trained how to integrate all of the information from the first three steps into one new rational response with the Rational Response Form (Handout 5.4 in Chapter 5), and how to check out their new interpretations through hypothesis testing. The Rational Response Form helps clients generate more adaptive thoughts, assumptions, and beliefs in a self-directed format. Hypothesis testing involves setting up real-life behavioral experiments that provide concrete data for evaluating the validity of different cognitive responses. In these experiments, the client is instructed to try out various alternative interpretations from the CR exercises and the behaviors that are consistent with these interpretations. Outcomes of these experiments are examined for evidence that either supports or refutes specific images, thoughts, assumptions, and beliefs.

Positive imagery purposefully replaces negative images evoked by particular stimulus events with realistic positive images. This includes imaging effective coping. This technique is based upon the principle of reciprocal inhibition (which also underlies the relaxation techniques discussed later). Reciprocal inhibition follows from the fact that parasympathetic and sympathetic activities of the autonomic nervous system are mutually exclusive. In other words, sensory images that activate parasympathetic activity can be used to counteract sensory images that activate sympathetic activity. This process strengthens associations of positive sensory imagery (and thereby parasympathetic activity) with stimulus events.

Worry exposure (Craske, Barlow, & O'Leary, 1992; Zinbarg, Craske, & Barlow, 1993) is used to confront cognitive avoidance of affective images. Worry exposure helps the client tolerate and accept, rather than avoid, unpleasant somatic sensations associated with affective images. Purposeful prolonged exposures to affective images enable habituation to somatic sensations and allow for conscious processing of any lack of congruence between affective images and environmental stimulus events. Successful outcomes of exposures are evident when disturbing images are viewed simply as disturbing images, not necessarily as representations of one's immediate context or vital interests.

Improving problem orientation (Dugas, Gagnon, Ladouceur, & Freeston, 1998) involves identifying key elements of a problem, while tolerating and coping with uncertain outcomes. This technique has two steps. The first focuses on identifying key elements of a problem by differentiating major from minor details and probable from improbable threats. The second requires clients to execute problem-solving behaviors only for major and probable threats, while learning to tolerate and cope with uncertainty.

Cost–benefit analysis of coping gives clients a structured way to evaluate the utility of various cognitive and/or behavioral coping responses. CR exercises are often incorporated in this analysis.

Two cognitive response prevention techniques—scheduled worry time (Borkovec, Wilkinson, Folensbee, & Lerner, 1983) and worry-free zones (Borkovec, Alcaine, & Behar, 2004)—interrupt and postpone the cognitive response of worry under certain stimulus conditions. With both of these techniques, clients are taught to select times and places where the cognitive response of worry is either prevented or permitted each day.

Scheduled worry time was originally conceived as a stimulus control technique. With this technique, the generalization of associations of worry with specific stimuli could be inhibited, and extinction could be promoted through tight restrictions on where and when worry was permitted. Borkovec et al. (2004) now describe the technique as a response prevention, albeit a cognitive response prevention, technique. Clients are taught to interrupt and postpone any activation of the cognitive response of worry (by "letting go" of worry) until the scheduled worry time.

Worry-free zones (Borkovec et al., 2004) are similar to Scheduled Worry time, except that certain times and locations are designated as worry-free periods. During those periods, worry is delayed or postponed. These worry-free zones are expanded over time.

The automatic cognitive response of worry to specific types of stimulus events can be extinguished with both of these techniques. The firm restrictions on where and when worry is allowed to occur can reduce the overall frequency and duration of worry episodes.

TECHNIQUES THAT TARGET THE PHYSIOLOGICAL COMPONENT

Excess physiological mobilization is addressed with techniques that utilize relaxation skills. Modified versions of Edmund Jacobson's progressive muscular relaxation (PMR) (Jacobson, 1928) and diaphragmatic breathing (DB) are skills that are taught to reduce symptoms of excess arousal. PMR exercises not only increase awareness of the location and degree of muscular tension, but provide a way of countering tension. DB increases awareness of problematic patterns of breathing that intensify and maintain physiological symptoms of arousal. DB allows the client to modify breathing patterns to resemble those that naturally occur in a relaxed state.

The two techniques that utilize relaxation skills are self-control desensitization (S-CD) and applied relaxation (AR). The S-CD technique (Goldfried, 1971) trains the client to engage in relaxation immediately upon recognition of any physiological mobilization during imaginal exposures to stimuli associated with worry. Opportunities to practice engaging in relaxation during imaginal exposures increase the client's ability to interrupt automatic associations and circumvent the spiraling process of worry. The AR technique (Öst, 1987) trains the client to apply relaxation across a wide variety of situations in daily life. In essence, both techniques allow the client to practice relaxation skills systematically in a variety of situations that evoke worry. These techniques increase the client's ability to interrupt physiological mobilization and any associated processes to circumvent the spiraling process of worry.

TECHNIQUES THAT TARGET THE BEHAVIORAL COMPONENT

Behavioral responses are modulated with techniques that include behavioral response prevention (Foa & Kozak, 1986), graded *in vivo* exposure, and pleasurable activity scheduling. Recent research (Schut, Castonguay, & Borkovec, 2001) indicates that compulsive checking is a relatively common compulsive behavior associated with GAD. Response prevention exercises reduce this and other excessive coping behaviors, such as preparatory, reassurance-seeking, overcautious, and/or protective behaviors, by teaching clients to resist engaging in these behaviors. The lack of consequences following exercises provides evidence to clients that these behaviors lack utility. Graded *in vivo* exposure is used to counter avoidance behaviors, including procrastination. Clients are taught to break down avoided situations into small steps and to approach those situations gradually, one step at a time. Graded *in vivo* exposure allows the client to build a sense of mastery and confidence with such situations. Pleasurable activity scheduling consists of identifying, planning, and scheduling pleasurable activities that have been delayed, postponed, forsaken, or avoided as the result of excessive and difficult-to-control worry.

TECHNIQUES THAT TARGET ASSOCIATED PROBLEMS

Other techniques that target problems potentially related to the worry process include mindfulness, emotional processing and regulation training, interpersonal effectiveness, and time management. Mindfulness (Roemer & Orsillo, 2002) counters tendencies toward experiential avoidance by strengthening awareness of the here-and-now. Emotional processing and regulation training (Mennin, Heimberg, Turk, & Fresco, 2002) increases awareness of one's emotional experience and provides alternatives to worry for regulating that emotional experience. Interpersonal effectiveness (Newman, Castonguay, Borkovec, & Molnar, 2004) increases awareness of habitual patterns of interaction that exacerbate and/or maintain symptoms, and provides ways to maximize the probability that one's personal needs and wants will be met with others. Time management (Craske et al., 1992; Roemer & Orsillo, 2002) focuses on identifying activities congruent with one's values and personal life goals, and planning and scheduling activities according to those priorities, while letting go of activities that are not consistent with those priorities.

EMPIRICAL SUPPORT FOR TREATMENT TECHNIQUES

Studies on various versions of cognitive-behavioral therapy (CBT) for GAD have provided strong support for the following techniques: CR, hypothesis testing, PMR, DB, S-CD, and AR. Since these techniques have received the strongest empirical support to date, they receive the most discussion in this book. There are relatively few studies on the following techniques, although they are potentially clinically useful: improving problem orientation, worry exposure, mindfulness, response prevention (cognitive and behavioral), *in vivo* exposure, pleasurable activity scheduling, time management, and positive imagery. More research is required to confirm the effectiveness of these techniques with GAD. Research on the techniques of interpersonal effectiveness and emotional processing and regulation training with difficult-to-treat clients is in progress, and outcome results are not yet available. If the therapist chooses to incorporate any of these latter techniques within a treatment package, it should be done with these cautions in mind.

BASICS OF IMPLEMENTING CBT TECHNIQUES

Effective implementation of these techniques requires a basic understanding of the principles of CBT, as well as skills in establishing positive rapport with clients and encouraging a collaborative relationship and a self-help attitude. The effective use of client forms is also an important aspect of treatment.

Building and Maintaining Positive Rapport

A positive therapeutic relationship is an essential ingredient in CBT. To build and maintain positive rapport between therapist and client, the therapist must be genuinely supportive and empathic with the client throughout treatment. This stance maximizes the chances that the client will feel cared for and understood by his or her therapist. It facilitates trust in the relationship and enhances motivation. This therapeutic stance is especially important when the therapist is confronting the client's cognitive distortions and maladaptive behaviors. Without such a relationship, the client is likely to feel defensive and will not be receptive to change.

Collaboration

The nature of the relationship between the therapist and client is collaborative. Together, they work as a team toward mutually agreed-upon goals. The therapist's role within this team is similar to that of a coach. The therapist works with the client to identify problems and teaches the client various techniques to manage problems and reduce symptoms. The client must be willing to take an active role in goal setting, self-monitoring, and experimenting with recommended treatment techniques. Without active client participation from the beginning, treatment is unlikely to succeed.

Encouraging a Self-Help Attitude

At the beginning of treatment, therapist participation is very important. The therapist must be actively involved in teaching the client each technique and helping the client discern ways techniques can be applied in everyday life. The therapist provides between-session assignments to help the client master techniques and discover positive outcomes from their applications. As treatment progresses, the client is encouraged to take increasing levels of responsibility for his or her own progress. This is accomplished by having the client generate more and more between-session assignments. The ultimate goal of this process is to teach the client how to continue utilizing treatment strategies independently of the therapist, so that the client's progress continues beyond therapy. The potency of treatment is largely dependent upon the client's willingness and ability to continue applying the techniques learned in treatment.

Using Client Forms

Clients are asked to fill out various forms throughout the course of this treatment. There are many purposes for the use of these forms or tracking records. As assessment tools (discussed in Chapter 3), they provide valuable information for identifying what to target in treatment and for measuring treatment effect and compliance. They are also used as treatment tools. First, records help to maintain a client's focus on the objectives of treatment between sessions. Second, record keeping increases the client's awareness of processes that typically occur on an automatic level and thus go unnoticed, thereby not allowing the client to intervene. The use of records helps the client gain distance from these processes and provides a stage for deliberately evaluating and altering them.

Therapists are encouraged to use the forms in this book in a flexible manner to meet the specific needs of their clients, or to develop their own forms when necessary. Some of the ways these forms can be used for assessment, treatment planning, and evaluation are described in Chapter 3. Chapters 5, 6, 7, and 8 demonstrate how they may be used as tools in treatment.

The following factors can increase client compliance with using the forms. The instructions about forms should be clear and concise. The therapist should give demonstrations and examples of how to fill out forms. The foci of forms should be limited to the specific targets in each client's treatment. The therapist should reinforce the client for record keeping by reiterating the benefits and praising compliance. The forms should be used to illustrate therapeutic change.

Because of its many benefits, client record keeping is strongly recommended. Some factors, however, may interfere with record keeping. These factors include illiteracy or learning disabilities. Specific types of record keeping may not be possible in certain settings, such as work settings where privacy is lacking. Although record keeping is not essential for therapeutic change, it can strengthen and speed the process of change.

Format of Treatment Sessions and Length of Treatment

The following session format is suggested to maintain the goal-directed focus within each 45- to 50-minute treatment session:

1. Develop an agenda for the session that includes specific treatment goals.
2. Review the main concepts from the prior session.
3. Review the client's progress with assignments from the prior session.
4. Complete the session's goals.
5. Assign self-help exercises to facilitate generalization of skills.
6. Conduct a session review.

Existing research suggests that 16–20 weekly sessions are adequate for standard CBT. Lengthening treatment with these techniques has not been found to improve treatment response (Newman, 2000). Given that the high-end-state recovery rates for the standard forms of CBT are 50%–60%, additional treatment with other techniques may be necessary. The needs of the client may require flexibility in terms of additional techniques and duration of treatment. As with all forms of CBT, full remission may not be possible in most cases. Rather, the goal is to equip the client sufficiently to continue the recovery process independently.

The next chapter discusses initial assessment of GAD, including the range of possible methods. The chapter then turns to treatment planning and details of session format and session length.

CHAPTER THREE

Assessment and Treatment Planning

Thorough assessments are critical for determining the existence and nature of GAD, planning appropriate treatment, and evaluating treatment outcome. There are three types of assessments. One type establishes the existence of GAD through a clinical interview format. Another establishes the existence and severity of the disorder through self-report measures. The last reveals, through both interview and self-report, how the disorder is expressed within a particular client's life; this third type accesses important information used in the planning and execution of treatment. All three types of assessments provide necessary data for comparing responses to treatment interventions with the pretreatment condition of GAD. Table 3.1 summarizes the possible methods for gathering these types of data.

DIAGNOSTIC CLINICAL INTERVIEWS

Clinical interviews with the purpose of establishing GAD as the primary diagnosis can be conducted in either a highly or a loosely structured manner. We discuss two highly structured empirically validated clinical interviews, and we give guidance for conducting loosely structured clinical interviews.

Highly Structured Clinical Interviews

There are a couple of advantages to using highly structured clinical interviews to assess GAD. First, accidental omissions from such an interview are less likely. Second, when conditions of the interview are held constant, comparisons of the disorder (pre- and posttreatment) are likely to reflect a change in the disorder, rather than a change in the way the disorder was assessed. The dis-

TABLE 3.1. Overview of Possible GAD Assessment Methods

Diagnostic clinical interviews
    Highly structured
        Anxiety Disorders Interview Schedule for DSM-IV (ADIS-IV)
        Structured Clinical Interview for DSM-IV (SCID)
    Loosely structured
        Decision Tree for Differential Diagnosis of GAD (Table 3.2)
        Decision Tree for GAD Diagnostic Criteria (Table 3.3)

Self-report measures for diagnosis and severity
    Beck Anxiety Inventory (BAI)
    Beck Depression Inventory-II (BDI-II)
    Penn State Worry Questionnaire (PSWQ)
    Generalized Anxiety Disorder Questionnaire—IV (GADQ-IV)

Assessing idiosyncratic aspects of GAD
    Life context interview
    Self-monitoring tools
        Worry Diary (Handout 3.1)
        Worry Episode Log (for Assessment) (Handout 3.2)

Assessing problematic patterns in relationships
    Inventory of Interpersonal Problems Circumplex Scales (IIP-C)
    Looking for patterns across client's relationships
    Exploring one relationship in depth
    Using therapist's emotional experiences with client to identify treatment targets

Assessing pleasurable activity
    Pleasurable Activity Log

advantage is that the interview can feel impersonal and awkward if the interviewer is not well familiarized with an instrument. The research-based structured clinical interviews that can be used to assess GAD are the Anxiety Disorders Interview Schedule for DSM-IV (ADIS-IV; DiNardo, Brown, & Barlow, 1994) and the Structured Clinical Interview for DSM-IV (SCID; First, Spitzer, Gibbon, & Williams, 1996, 1997).

The ADIS-IV (DiNardo, 1994)[1] is an empirically validated and reliable structured clinical interview that is particularly advantageous for differentiating GAD from other anxiety disorders. The ADIS-IV provides in-depth assessment of adult anxiety, mood, and substance-related disorders, as well as two somatoform disorders (hypochrondriasis and somatization disorder). The ADIS-IV also provides quick screening for psychotic disorders. There are several short versions for follow-up assessments.

The SCID (First et al., 1996, 1997)[2] can also be used to conduct an empirically validated and reliable structured clinical interview. The advantage of the SCID is that it is more comprehensive than the ADIS-IV, in that all adult disorders can be assessed. The Clinical Version of the SCID

---

[1]The ADIS-IV is available at *www.PsychCorp.com*.
[2]The SCID is available at *www.appi.org*. Information about the SCID is available at *www.scid4.org*.

(SCID-CV) is used to assess Axis I disorders, and the SCID for Personality Disorders (SCID-II) is used to assess Axis II disorders.

Loosely Structured Clinical Interview

It is likely that loosely structured clinical interviews are the most common means by which therapists in outpatient and private-practice settings conduct initial diagnostic assessments. Table 3.2 provides questions for ruling out other possible diagnoses and ensuring that a client's symptoms meet criteria for GAD, when anxiety is presented as the initial complaint.

If the answers to the questions in Table 3.2 are no, then the therapist should assess for GAD by considering the questions in Table 3.3. All of these questions require a positive response for a diagnosis of GAD. If responses are partially positive, a diagnosis of anxiety disorder not otherwise specified (NOS) may be considered.

The following clinical vignette shows the diagnostic portion of a loosely structured assessment interview. Richard is a tall, thin, and relatively handsome 32-year-old man. As he speaks, his face appears drawn and tense. Richard sits erect, leaning slightly forward on the couch. He kneads and tightly clenches his hands, and he shifts position frequently. As he speaks, he periodically takes in large breaths (as if trying to catch his breath) and sighs repeatedly. The therapist observes that the client's statements and body language indicate restlessness and muscle tension.

> THERAPIST: What brings you here today?
>
> CLIENT: I made this appointment because of my wife. She thinks I'm a nervous wreck. I agree with her, but frankly, Doctor, I don't know if I have time for this. I have so much pressure on me. I never can relax. I really shouldn't be taking the time for this. It's too self-indulgent. I have enormous responsibilities at work and at home. Everyone's depending on me. I really don't think I can handle all of this.
>
> THERAPIST: It sounds like you're feeling overwhelmed by the prospect of therapy on top of all of your other responsibilities. Is that right? [Therapist expresses empathy, laying foundation for rapport.]
>
> CLIENT: Yes. That's right.
>
> THERAPIST: If we take therapy out of the picture, how often do you have these feelings of nervousness, being unable to relax, under pressure, and overwhelmed by your responsibilities? [Assessing frequency of anxiety or stress response]
>
> CLIENT: I feel this way most of the time. My family complains that I'm working or distracted most of the time and not paying attention to them. I can't stop thinking about all the things I have to do at work. I'm constantly worried that I missed something or screwed up something. [Therapist notices that the client's statements indicate worry and difficulty controlling worry, but checks this observation with the client.]
>
> THERAPIST: It sounds like you spend a lot of time worrying about your work performance, and it's hard for you to stop worrying.
>
> CLIENT: Yes. I worry a lot!

TABLE 3.2. Decision Tree for Differential Diagnosis of GAD

Is the anxiety related to embarrassment or humiliation in social situations?

    NO   YES—assess for social phobia

Have there been any sudden rushes of anxiety for no apparent reason?

    NO   YES—assess for panic disorder and agoraphobia

Is there persistent fear of a specific object or situation?

    NO   YES—assess for specific phobia

Has there been exposure to a traumatic event?

    NO   YES—assess for posttraumatic stress disorder or acute stress disorder

Is the anxiety associated with recurrent and intrusive images that do not make sense to the client? Does the client engage in repetitive behaviors or thoughts to lessen uncomfortable feelings?

    NO   YES—assess for obsessive–compulsive disorder

Is the anxiety restricted to loss of or separation from a significant other or from home, and was the onset before 18 years of age?

    NO   YES—assess for separation anxiety disorder

Is there persistent fear of serious disease or illness that has been medically evaluated and not supported?

    NO   YES—assess for hypochrondriasis

Are there physical complaints (e.g., fatigue, gastrointestinal problems, or urinary problems) that cannot be fully explained by, or are in excess of, a known medical condition?

    NO   YES—assess for somatization disorder or undifferentiated somatoform disorder

Is there persistent fear about gaining weight, accompanied by underweight appearance?

    NO   YES—assess for anorexia nervosa

Is there preoccupation with a perceived defect in appearance that is markedly excessive?

    NO   YES—assess for body dysmorphic disorder

Did the symptoms occur within 3 months of the onset of an identifiable stressor, and is the stressor still present?

    NO   YES—assess for adjustment disorder with anxiety

Is there a medical condition that could account for the anxiety?

    NO   YES—assess for anxiety disorder due to a general medical condition

Can the anxiety be attributed to a drug, medication, or toxin?

    NO   YES—assess for substance-induced anxiety disorder

Does the anxiety occur exclusively during the course of a mood disorder?

    NO   YES—assess for mood disorders

Does the anxiety occur exclusively during the course of a psychotic disorder?

    NO   YES—assess for psychotic disorders

TABLE 3.3. Decision Tree for GAD Diagnostic Criteria

Are the anxiety and worry about a number of events or activities?

Are the anxiety and worry excessive?

Is the worry difficult to control?

Do the anxiety and worry occur more days than not?

Have they been present for at least 6 months?

Have three or more of the following symptoms been present to some degree over the last 6 months (one symptom, if the client is a child):
- Restless, keyed up, on edge
- Easily fatigued
- Difficulty concentrating or mind going blank
- Irritable
- Muscle tension
- Disturbed sleep

Does the anxiety, worry, or physical symptoms cause clinically significant distress or interference with functioning (daily routine, social, or occupational)?

From *Treating Generalized Anxiety Disorder* by Jayne L. Rygh and William C. Sanderson. Copyright 2004 by The Guilford Press. Permission to photocopy this table is granted to purchasers of this book for personal use only (see copyright page for details).

THERAPIST: What is it about your performance that you are worried about? Are you worried about embarrassing or humiliating yourself in front of others, or is it something else? [Assessing for social phobia]

CLIENT: I'm worried that I'm going to lose my job. Getting fired would be embarrassing, but that's not what I'm worried about. I'm worried I won't be able to support my family, and we'll end up out on the street.

THERAPIST: Are there other things that you worry about? [Assessing the foci of worry]

CLIENT: Sometimes I worry about my health. Sometimes I worry that something terrible will happen to my kids.

THERAPIST: What about your health? [Assessing for hypochrondriasis, somatization disorder, and undifferentiated somatoform disorder]

CLIENT: I'm worried that I'm going to cause my body to break down from all this stress and worry.

THERAPIST: Have you gone to the doctor with a variety of problems over the years? [Assessing for somatization disorder]

CLIENT: In the past, I went a couple of times outside of my regular checkups.

THERAPIST: What was that for?

CLIENT: One time I was worried that I had cancer. Another time I was worried that I was having symptoms of a heart attack.

THERAPIST: How long were you concerned about these things? [Assessing for undifferentiated somatoform disorder]

CLIENT: I remember that I had this spot on my skin, and I was worried for a few weeks that it meant that I had cancer. The other time I kept noticing this feeling of tightness in my chest. That lasted about a month. I thought I was having symptoms of a heart attack. Both times I went to the doctor.

THERAPIST: And what happened?

CLIENT: My doctor told me I was in good health. He told me that my anxiety was the problem.

THERAPIST: Did you continue to believe that you had cancer or were at risk for heart attack, despite the doctor's reassurance? [Assessing for hypochondriasis]

CLIENT: No. I was able to stop worrying about those specific things, but I still worry that I'm going to cause some kind of health problem with all this stress and worry.

THERAPIST: You mentioned you worry about your kids.

CLIENT: Yes. When I take them to a park or even at home, I worry something terrible will happen.

THERAPIST: Like . . .

CLIENT: I get images of one of them getting hit by a car while crossing the street to the park, or falling off the playground equipment and being paralyzed. Just talking about it makes me anxious.

THERAPIST: Do these images and thoughts seem realistic to you? [Assessing for obsessive–compulsive disorder]

CLIENT: Sure. Accidents happen.

THERAPIST: Do you do anything when these images occur?

CLIENT: I hold on tight to my kids when we cross the street. Sometimes I think of something other than going to the playground that doesn't involve any risk.

THERAPIST: Have you ever experienced or witnessed a traumatic or life-threatening event, like seeing someone badly hurt or killed, an assault, a natural or a human-made disaster? [Assessing for posttraumatic stress disorder]

CLIENT: No. Thank goodness.

THERAPIST: Earlier, you said you feel this way most of the time. Do you feel this way more days than not? [Assessing for GAD criteria]

CLIENT: Definitely.

THERAPIST: You also said that your family complains that you're working or distracted most of the time and not paying attention to them. Do you find it difficult to control your worry about work, your kids, and your health? [Assessing for GAD criteria]

CLIENT: Yes, I would say so.

THERAPIST: Do you think you worry more than necessary? In other words, do you find yourself worrying at times when it is not productive, like during the night when it would be better to sleep? [Assessing for GAD criteria]

CLIENT: Yes. That happens a lot.

THERAPIST: How long has worry been interfering with your life? [Assessing for GAD criteria]

CLIENT: I think I've always been a worrier, but it's been much worse over the last 4 years.

THERAPIST: Was there a change or difficult circumstance that occurred around that time? [Assessing for adjustment disorder]

CLIENT: Well, I started the job that I have now around that time.

THERAPIST: And what was it like when you started?

CLIENT: When I started with this firm, I had this boss who demanded perfection, even when deadlines were unbelievably tight. She was a constant bug about productivity. She expected every minute to be utilized in the most efficient way.

THERAPIST: Is she still there?

CLIENT: No. She left the firm about a year and a half ago.

THERAPIST: And how is your current boss?

CLIENT: He's much more reasonable. Even though my current boss is a nice guy, I still worry about how I'm doing. I can't seem to stop these worries. On the weekends, if I see my briefcase or work shoes or if I hear something on the radio related to work, I start worrying. My wife is right—it is out of hand.

THERAPIST: Are there any other problems that you're experiencing? [Open probe for other presenting problems]

CLIENT: Yes. You said something about worrying instead of sleeping. My sleep is not great. Several nights a week, I wake up in the middle of the night and have trouble going back to sleep because I start worrying about something. I feel exhausted all the time. [Since client's primary complaints are related to GAD, and GAD criteria are met, sleep disorders are ruled out.]

THERAPIST: Are you having any other problems?

CLIENT: Not really.

THERAPIST: What about your mood? How has your mood been? [Assessing for mood disorders]

CLIENT: Off and on, I feel a little down.

THERAPIST: How often do you feel that way?

CLIENT: I feel that way for a day or two, usually a couple times a month. Most of the time I feel OK. The main problem is this anxiety.

THERAPIST: Do you ever experience sudden rushes of intense fear or feelings of impending doom? [Assessing for panic disorder]

CLIENT: Sometimes I feel panicked, if that's what you're asking.

THERAPIST: Have those feelings ever come from out of the blue, for no apparent reason?

CLIENT: No. But, I've gotten those feelings when I'm really worried about something.

THERAPIST: The anxiety that you're experiencing, have you found anything that gives you relief? [Assessing for substance abuse or dependence]

CLIENT: On the weekends, I have a Scotch before dinner. That gives me a little relief.

THERAPIST: How many shots of Scotch do you have?

CLIENT: My wife fixes the drink. I think she gives me an ounce and a half.

THERAPIST: Do you ever drink more than that?

CLIENT: Back in college and law school, I got drunk a few times. But I don't let myself drink like that now. I have too many responsibilities. Also, I'm worried it could become a problem if I let myself go. I want to find other ways to relieve my anxiety. I'm not in the market for a drinking problem on top of my anxiety problems.

THERAPIST: What about other substances, like recreational drugs or taking a prescription at a higher dose than prescribed?

CLIENT: No, thanks. That stuff never was for me.

THERAPIST: How about over-the-counter remedies, like herbs?

CLIENT: No.

THERAPIST: Do you drink much caffeine?

CLIENT: One cup of coffee in the morning and one cup in the early afternoon. I get the shakes if I drink more than that.

THERAPIST: Have you been exposed to any toxic substances? [Ruling out anxiety resulting from exposure to toxins]

CLIENT: Nothing more than the usual toxic fumes in the city.

THERAPIST: Going back to something you said in the beginning, you mentioned that there's some tension in your relationship with your wife.

CLIENT: Yes, she's frustrated that I'm not able to spend more time with her and the family.

THERAPIST: How are your relationships in general? [Assessing for personality disorder]

CLIENT: Overall, I think my wife and I have a pretty good relationship. We have our problems, but we seem to be able to work most of them out. We have a lot of good friends, but we don't see them enough. I don't feel like I see enough of my kids, either. That bothers me a lot. The main problem is this anxiety.

In this vignette, the therapist observes the client's behavior and follows up the client's statements with specific questions that are aimed at clarifying the nature of the symptoms. As many clients with GAD do, Richard states early in the interview that difficult-to-control worry is a problem for him. The therapist poses a number of questions regarding the foci of worry to determine whether the primary disorder is GAD, another anxiety disorder, or a disorder of another type. In addition, questions about the frequency, intensity, and duration of worry; difficulties with controlling worry; and distress and impairment associated with worry are asked to determine whether criteria for GAD are met. The circumstances associated with the onset and duration of the disorder are explored to rule out the possibility that the symptoms are due to external circumstances, such as a highly stressful event, ingestion of a substance, or exposure to a toxin. Additional questions that probe for common coexisting disorders, such as mood disorders, substance abuse or dependence, and personality disorders, ensure that the assessment is comprehensive.

SELF-REPORT MEASURES FOR DIAGNOSIS AND SEVERITY

Four empirically validated and reliable self-report measures can be used for quick assessments of anxiety, depression, worry, and GAD. These are the Beck Anxiety Inventory (BAI; Beck, Epstein, Brown, & Steer, 1988),[3] the Beck Depression Inventory—II (BDI-II; Beck, Steer, & Brown, 1996), the Penn State Worry Questionnaire (PSWQ; Meyer, Miller, Metzger, & Borkovec, 1990),[4] and the Generalized Anxiety Disorder Questionnaire—IV (GADQ-IV; Newman et al., 2002).

The BAI is a 21-item self-report measure of general anxiety (somatic and psychological symptoms). General anxious arousal is an essential feature of GAD. The BAI scores range from 0 to 63. Steer, Clark, Beck, and Ranieri (1999) found patients with a principal diagnosis of GAD ($n = 151$) obtained a mean score of 19.95 ($SD = 10.86$) on this scale.

The BDI-II is a 21-item self-report measure for assessing the intensity of depression. Testing on a large clinical population ($n = 500$) demonstrated high reliability (coefficient alpha $= .92$) (Steer, Brown, Beck, & Sanderson, 1999).

The PSWQ is a 16-item questionnaire used to measure worry. It was designed to discriminate individuals with GAD from those with other anxiety disorders (Brown, Antony, & Barlow, 1992). The internal consistency of the measure is good (.91). The measure also has good convergent and discriminant validity (Meyer et al., 1990). Molina and Borkovec (1994) found the mean score of patients with GAD ($n = 174$) to be 67.66 ($SD = 8.86$). Using a French version of the PSWQ, Dupuy, Beaudoin, Rheaume, Ladouceur, and Dugas (2001) compared GAD diagnosed individuals with a nonclinical population. They found that the population with GAD obtained a mean score of 62.18 ($SD = 7.9$), in contrast to the nonclinical population's mean score of 41.08 ($SD = 9.4$).

The GADQ-IV is a revised self-report diagnostic measure of GAD based on the DSM-IV criteria. Preliminary data (Newman et al., 2002) on the GADQ-IV showed 89% specificity and 83% sensitivity when compared to highly structured interview diagnoses of individuals with GAD. The self-report measure demonstrated test–retest reliability, convergent and discriminant validity, and kappa agreement of .67 with a highly structured interview.

The therapist may choose to include other types of self-report assessment tools as well. Other areas for assessment might include marital/couple functioning and/or social functioning.

ASSESSING IDIOSYNCRATIC ASPECTS OF GAD

Once the client's primary diagnosis is established as GAD, the therapist can begin to gain more intimate knowledge of how the disorder is expressed within the client's life. This is accomplished first by broadly learning about the course of the disorder over the client's life span, and then by

---

[3] The Beck scales are available at *www.PsychCorp.com*.
[4] The PSWQ is available at *www.tdb@mail.psu.edu*.

closely examining various aspects of the client's worry. The information from this part of the assessment is used later to determine a specific treatment plan for the individual client.

Life Context Interview

A life context interview should cover the following issues in regard to the client's anxiety:

- Onset circumstances
- Duration
- Course
- Life events associated with exacerbations
- Coping efforts
- Previous treatments

First, of course, understanding GAD over the client's life span includes learning about the onset, duration, and course of the disorder. Life events associated with exacerbations of the disorder indicate vulnerable points to be fortified. Investigating the client's efforts to cope with GAD can reveal successful strategies to be built upon and/or problematic strategies to be eliminated. Finally, exploring previous treatments of the disorder can highlight specific problems with particular techniques in terms of frequency of usage, focus of attention, and/or persistence.

The following clinical vignette continues Richard's assessment interview. The therapist now turns to learning about the issues listed above in the context of Richard's life.

THERAPIST: When did you first notice that worry was a problem?

CLIENT: Well, I've been a worrier for as long as I can remember. I know it definitely got worse when I took this job right after my son was born, 4 years ago.

THERAPIST: Yes, you mentioned that earlier. Have you ever had any periods like this before?

CLIENT: I guess I did, come to think of it. Actually, there's been quite a few.

THERAPIST: What are you remembering?

CLIENT: I remember my mom saying that I was extremely anxious when I was in elementary school. I know I had a lot of anxiety through most of my school years.

THERAPIST: Do you remember any changes or difficulties that occurred around the times that the anxiety started or got worse?

CLIENT: We moved to a new neighborhood right before I started elementary school, but I don't remember much about that period of time. I was only 4 years old. At the start of junior high. . . . I remember worrying a lot and feeling generally insecure. I had been put in private school, instead of continuing public school with my best friend. College and law school were stressful, especially law school. Right before I started law school, my cousin, with whom I was close, was killed in an auto accident.

THERAPIST: Do you remember what you worried about during any of those periods?

CLIENT: I guess I've always worried about whether I'm doing well enough—in school, and now at work. After my cousin's death, I remember that I started worrying that something really horrible could happen without warning. Those worries have lasted most of my life.

THERAPIST: Do you remember any periods of time when you stopped worrying?

CLIENT: In elementary school . . . the only time I remember feeling relaxed was in fifth grade, after I met my friend Scott. He was the total opposite of me. He was the class clown—took nothing seriously. I remember having a great time cutting up with him in class, but I got into a lot of trouble with him. I remember my parents getting furious about my behavior and school performance, and that bothering me. But I also remember the temptation to have fun with Scott was something I couldn't resist. The fun ended with elementary school. My parents put me in private school in sixth grade. Although my parents never admitted it, I think they changed my school to separate us. I never saw Scott after that, and I went right back to my anxious self.

I remember feeling anxious through junior high and most of high school . . . I remember feeling better towards the end of senior year. Maybe that was because the pressure was off after I was accepted in college. I remember feeling free, no worries or responsibilities. That time was great, but it didn't last long—only about 6 months.

I was always worried in college . . . about my grades, figuring out my major and what I was going to do with my life. And law school . . . more of the same.

Law school was hell. After I finished, I desperately needed a break. I just took off after my last exam and traveled aimlessly for about a year. I guess I felt like it was my last gasp of freedom before the serious business of life. I paid for that break later, though. I had a hard time finding work when I came back. I guess I didn't look serious to employers after a year's vacation. None of my classmates did what I did. They all went into jobs either immediately or after a brief break.

THERAPIST: It sounds like you've coped with these intense anxiety-ridden periods by indulging yourself with equally intense periods of pleasure. Is that right?

CLIENT: Yes. That was true in the past. I don't have that option now.

THERAPIST: Have you found any other ways of relieving your worry and anxiety?

CLIENT: It seems that working is the only thing that gives me any relief. I can't just blow things off now. . . . I used to exercise before the kids were born. That helped. I have trouble finding the time now. I just have too many responsibilities.

THERAPIST: What about therapy? Have you ever been in therapy before?

CLIENT: No. But, I did go to a stress management group sponsored at work.

THERAPIST: What was that like?

CLIENT: They did this relaxation exercise, which was good. I did feel relaxed during the exercise, but I felt worse later.

THERAPIST: What happened?

CLIENT: After I got back to my office, I got worried that taking that much time off from work every day would make me feel even more stressed. So I only went once.

From this interaction, the therapist learns several things. The disorder has been long-standing, with a few short remissions. Remissions only occurred when the client "blew things off" or escaped from his usual activities and responsibilities. Onset and/or exacerbations of symptoms were associated with major life events (move, change of schools or job, cousin's death). This indicates that stressful life events are likely to exacerbate Richard's symptoms or increase the probability of relapse, if not addressed in treatment. The only current coping strategy to reduce anxiety is overworking. This strategy effectively reduces anxiety in the short term, but is ineffective for long-term reduction of anxiety. No prior treatment has been sought, with the exception of one session of relaxation training. Although the client was able to achieve a relaxed state in this one session, the prior problems with follow-through would need to be addressed with the reintroduction of this technique.

Self-Monitoring Tools

The client's worry can be assessed in detail in two different ways. First, worry can be examined on a daily basis with respect to frequency and intensity. Second, each episode of worry can be examined in terms of stimulus triggers, duration, and associated elements (cognitive, physiological, and behavioral). The Worry Diary captures the first type of information, and the Worry Episode Log (for Assessment) garners the second. The Worry Episode Log is particularly important for identifying specific targets for treatment. In addition to worry, individuals with GAD often present with deficits in pleasurable activity. The Pleasurable Activity Log can be used to assess the amount of pleasurable activity in daily life. Clients are asked to begin keeping records with these forms in the assessment phase of treatment (Session 1 and/or Session 2) and are instructed to continue throughout the treatment phase. When these records are used throughout the treatment phase, they provide data for determining treatment compliance and the degree of change over the course of treatment.

Worry Diary

The Worry Diary (see Handout 3.1) is a quick and easy tool that is used to obtain information about worry each day over the course of a week. The client is asked to enter several different types of information about worry every day. The first type is to rate the percentage (0%–100%) of the day spent in worry (excluding time asleep). The second is to rate the overall intensity of anxiety (on a scale of 0–8) experienced throughout the day. The third is to record the number of minutes spent in worry during that day. The form also provides a section to record daily usage of medication for anxiety.

Two studies have provided reference points for the type of information collected with this form. Craske, Rapee, Jackel, and Barlow (1989) found that individuals diagnosed with GAD reported an average of 60.7% of the day worrying, while control subjects reported a daily average of 18.2%. Dupuy et al. (2001) compared the time spent worrying in individuals diagnosed with GAD with a nonclinical population. They found individuals with GAD spent 310 minutes ($SD = 195.5$), versus the nonclinical population's 55 minutes ($SD = 62.9$), in worry each day.

It is ideal if the client fills out the diary each day and brings the diary to each session. The diary gives the therapist a general overview of the degree of interference from worry on a weekly

WORRY DIARY

Instructions: Use a separate line for each day of the week. On each line, fill out the date, make three estimates, and record any medication usage. The three estimates are as follows: (1) What percentage (0%–100%) of that day (waking hours) was spent in worry? (2) What was your overall level of anxiety on that day (use the 0–8 anxiety scale)? (3) How many minutes did you spend in worry that day?

Anxiety scale

0	1	2	3	4	5	6	7	8
None		Mild		Moderate		Severe		Extreme

Date	Percent of day worried (0%–100%)	Overall anxiety (0–8 scale)	Minutes worried	Medications (type/dosage)

basis. Changes over time are easily observed from the ratings for each week. The following vignette illustrates the therapist instructing the client on how to complete the form.

> THERAPIST: Richard, I want you to look at this form (*hands Worry Diary to client*) . . . As you can see, there are seven slots on this sheet, one for each day. Every day, I want you to make three estimates. One estimate is the percent of that day spent in worry. Another is to rate your overall level of anxiety on that day. The third is to estimate how many minutes you worried that day. Let's use today as an example of how to fill out this form. In this column, write today's day and date.
>
> CLIENT: OK.
>
> THERAPIST: Do you think you could estimate what percent of your day has been spent in worry today?
>
> CLIENT: (*Pause*) . . . I guess it's about 60%.
>
> THERAPIST: Write that down. And how would you rate your overall level of anxiety so far? Use this 0–8 scale, with 0 representing no anxiety, 2 as mild anxiety, 4 as moderate, 6 as severe, and 8 as extreme.
>
> CLIENT: Probably 6.
>
> THERAPIST: Write that down. And what is your best estimate of the number of minutes spent in worry today?
>
> CLIENT: (*Pause*) . . . Well, I worried some this morning. I felt worried before I got to work. That was about an hour. Then I worked fairly hard, except for about a half-hour in the morning. That was because I started to worry about taking time for this appointment.
>
> THERAPIST: That's 90 minutes . . . what about this afternoon and evening?
>
> CLIENT: I started to have a hard time getting work done after about 3:00, because I started worrying again about coming to this appointment. That basically lasted until I got here at 7:30. . . . So I guess that was another 270 minutes. Let's see, 270 + 90 = 360.
>
> THERAPIST: Write that down in this column. If you were on medication or taking an herbal supplement, you would put that information in this column. But you can ignore that column, since you are not taking anything. I want you to complete this form at the end of every day and bring this form with you to every session. This form will allow both of us to see if any changes are occurring with treatment.
>
> CLIENT: OK.

Figure 3.1 shows a Worry Diary completed by Richard for an entire week.

Worry Episode Log (for Assessment)

The assessment version of the Worry Episode Log (see Handout 3.2) heightens awareness (in both therapist and client) of the elements of worry in the individual client. Clear identification of all active individual components during episodes of worry illuminates specific points for treatment in-

WORRY DIARY

Instructions: Use a separate line for each day of the week. On each line, fill out the date, make three estimates, and record any medication usage. The three estimates are as follows: (1) What percentage (0%–100%) of that day (waking hours) was spent in worry? (2) What was your overall level of anxiety on that day (use the 0–8 anxiety scale)? (3) How many minutes did you spend in worry that day?

Anxiety scale								
0	1	2	3	4	5	6	7	8
None		Mild		Moderate		Severe		Extreme

Date	Percent of day worried (0%–100%)	Overall anxiety (0–8 scale)	Minutes worried	Medications (type/dosage)
2/20	75	7	620	none
2/21	55	5	510	none
2/22	60	6	585	none
2/23	45	4	425	none
2/24	58	6	545	none
2/25	70	7	605	none
2/26	60	6	520	none

FIGURE 3.1. Richard's Worry Diary.

tervention. In addition, the log can be used to create treatment hierarchies (as discussed in Chapter 7). A modified version of this log is used in the treatment phase and is discussed in Chapter 5.

Several important pieces of information should be filled out on this form in the assessment phase. The day, date, and time of the worry episode should be noted. Although the log can be completed in retrospect, this is not ideal; retrospective completion may not be as accurate as an immediate response, because recall biases increase with the passage of time. Internal and external stimuli (triggers) associated with the onset of worry are important to include. The intensity of anxiety, amount of control over worry, and the experience of any other emotions during the worry episode are to be recorded. Most important to note are the cognitive (images, thoughts, assumptions, and beliefs), physiological, and behavioral activities that occur during the episode of worry. Lastly, the duration of the episode is entered. The following clinical vignette provides an example of the therapist instructing the client on how to complete this form.

HANDOUT 3.2. Worry Episode Log (for Assessment)

WORRY EPISODE LOG (FOR ASSESSMENT)

Day/date/time of episode:

Circle maximum intensity of anxiety during worry episode.

0	1	2	3	4	5	6	7	8
None		Mild		Moderate		Severe		Extreme

Circle amount of control over worry episode.

0	1	2	3	4	5	6	7	8
None		Low		Moderate		High		Complete

Other emotions (e.g., anger, sadness, hurt . . . with intensity ratings):

Worry triggers (internal and/or external): What started the worry? _____

Mind: What is happening in your mind? (Rate how convincing on 0–8 scale: ___)

    Images: _____

    Thoughts, assumptions, beliefs (about self, others, situation, function of worry): _____

_____

_____

Body: How is your body responding physically? _____

_____

_____

Actions/behaviors: What do you do (or not do)? _____

_____

How long was the worry episode? _____

THERAPIST: Let's take your last episode of worry in hand. What was happening when you first noticed yourself worrying?

CLIENT: I was in my car, coming here. There was much more traffic than usual. I was feeling totally overwhelmed and distressed, thinking, "Oh, my God, I am going to be late."

THERAPIST: OK. So write down today's day, date, and the time of the episode on this form. I want you to rate the intensity of your anxiety or worry while you were in this situation. Using this 0–8 scale on the top of this sheet, with 0 representing no anxiety or worry, 2 representing a mild level, 4 as moderate, 6 as severe, and 8 as extreme, how would you rate what you felt at that time?

CLIENT: About 7.

THERAPIST: You were pretty anxious. OK. Circle the 7. How much control did you have over the worry in this situation?

CLIENT: What do you mean?

THERAPIST: Do you think you could have stopped yourself from worrying?

CLIENT: No. I was too anxious about getting here late.

THERAPIST: Try to rate the degree of control over worry, again using the 0–8 scale at the top of this sheet. 0 represents no control, and the numbers go up to 8. An 8 indicates complete control. How much control over worry did you feel in this situation?

CLIENT: I guess about 1.

THERAPIST: OK. Circle 1. Were you feeling any other emotions in this situation, like anger or sadness or any other emotion?

CLIENT: Maybe a bit of anger, because I have too much to do.

THERAPIST: OK. Write that emotion down and rate it on the 0–8 scale. . . . Do you remember what was happening when you noticed your anxiety beginning to rise?

CLIENT: (*Pause*) . . . The traffic started to get heavy, and it was slowing me down.

THERAPIST: Good. Write that down next to "Worry triggers." Did you have any images while this was occurring?

CLIENT: Yeah. I was imagining that you would be really angry about the lateness. I feel embarrassed telling you this. It sounds so ridiculous now. I should be able to handle these situations in a mature fashion without having to get help.

THERAPIST: I am really glad that you are telling me this. Feeling embarrassed about revealing what goes on inside of you during these times is something that I hear very frequently from clients at the initial stages of treatment. It sounds like part of you wants to hide and feels like you should be beyond this; yet another part of you is ready to risk exposing some of this stuff so that you can get help. I want to appeal to the side of you that is willing to take some risks. How about using this session as an experiment to see how you feel at the end of the session after taking the risk of exposing what's going on inside of you?

CLIENT: OK.

THERAPIST: So write down under "Mind," next to "Images," the image of an angry therapist. In therapy, we define "cognition" as any image, thought, assumption, or belief that runs through your mind. Sometimes these cognitive events occur very quickly and are difficult to catch. Did you notice anything else running through your mind at that time?

CLIENT: I assumed you'd tell me that I'm not a good candidate for therapy, given that I couldn't get here on time. I was thinking, "This whole situation is intolerable, because I have to get help." I also was thinking that I probably wasted time and put myself under even more intense pressure by coming here, rather than less.

THERAPIST: OK. Write all this down under "Mind," next to "Thoughts, assumptions, beliefs": "I assumed I would be told I was not a good candidate. I thought the situation was intolerable. I thought I probably wasted time and put myself under even more intense pressure."

THERAPIST: What kind of beliefs did you have about yourself when this was occurring?

CLIENT: (Pause) . . . I'm always making mistakes. Whatever I do is never good enough. I should have left earlier to make sure I got here on time.

THERAPIST: What about beliefs about others in relation to you?

CLIENT: I guess that mistakes are not OK. You get rejected if you don't behave correctly.

THERAPIST: What about beliefs about situations like this?

CLIENT: I guess that something is always going wrong. Life is so unpredictable.

THERAPIST: What do you believe about the process of worry in these types of situations? Why worry?

CLIENT: Worry keeps me more focused on what I'm doing. In this situation, I thought it would get me here faster. I also thought that you might be more forgiving of my tardiness if you saw how serious I was about getting here.

THERAPIST: Write those beliefs down next to your thoughts and assumptions. You can write, "Whatever I do is never good enough. I get rejected by others when I make mistakes. Life is unpredictable. Worry keeps me focused on what I'm doing. My worry makes others more forgiving of my mistakes." . . . At the time that all of this was occurring, how strongly did you believe these cognitions were true, on a 0–8 scale?

CLIENT: About 7.

THERAPIST: Write down that rating where it says "Rate how convincing . . . " in parentheses. (Pause) . . . It sounds like you were experiencing a lot of anxiety with those cognitions, which were very believable to you. What were the physical sensations or symptoms you were experiencing in this situation?

CLIENT: I was really tense. I think my chest felt tight. I was taking a lot of deep breaths.

THERAPIST: Were you breathing like this (demonstrates large breaths through the chest) or like this (demonstrates deep diaphragmatic breaths)?

CLIENT: Definitely the first.

THERAPIST: OK. Write down "Tense, tightness in chest, large chest breath" next to "Body." What were you doing in this situation?

CLIENT: I started checking the clock every 20 to 30 seconds. I started weaving in and out of traffic trying to get ahead. I was yelling at all the cars ahead of me. No one could hear me, of course, because I had the windows shut. I ran several yellow lights—actually, one had just turned red—on my way here. Fortunately, no cops were around.

THERAPIST: OK. Next to "Actions/behaviors," write down each of those behaviors. . . . It sounds like you were responding on a number of levels as if you were in an emergency situation.

CLIENT: Yeah. I was. I could have gotten a ticket or had an accident with the way I was driving.

THERAPIST: It sounds like you temporarily lost sight of the relative importance of different priorities—getting to this appointment on time, versus driving safely to prevent injury to yourself or others.

CLIENT: That definitely is true, and that kind of thing makes me even more worried. Looking back at how I was thinking and what I did, I really feel like I'm not in control at those times.

THERAPIST: The last section is for writing down the duration of the episode. How long did this episode last?

CLIENT: Well, I'm not sure. I got here on time, so that worry disappeared. But, I started worrying that you were going to think I was a real nut job once I got in here.

THERAPIST: OK. That sounds like an even more recent, but different, episode of worry. That worry would be recorded on a separate log sheet. When did you stop worrying about being late?

CLIENT: When I got here at 7:58 P.M.

THERAPIST: So this episode lasted how long?

CLIENT: I guess about 30 minutes.

THERAPIST: Write that down. . . . We just worked through this form retrospectively, and that can be helpful. The most helpful time to fill out this form, though, is during an episode of worry. The only item that must be done retrospectively is the duration of the episode. It is very important that you begin to record episodes of worry on copies of this form.

There are two advantages in filling out this form during an episode. First, observing and recording an episode will allow you to slow down and interrupt the process of worry. Right now, the process is occurring quickly and automatically. Sometimes the process may be so quick that you may miss some of the elements of worry. You may find that you have to really concentrate to catch what is occurring at these times. The benefit of careful recording is that the recording allows you to gain some distance from the worry. This distance will make it easier to recognize when and where you can implement techniques to reduce worry. You will be learning a variety of techniques for this purpose. Second, completing a copy of this form whenever you have a worry episode will speed up your treatment. The more quickly we can assess the problem areas, the sooner we can begin to systematically apply techniques in those areas.

I know that sometimes you won't be able to fill out this form during an episode. In those instances, try to record the episode retrospectively. If you do it retrospectively, carefully retrace the sequence of events as they occurred. Complete the form as soon as possible. The longer you wait, the more difficult it will be to remember accurately what happened during the episode.

Your assignment for next week is to fill out the Worry Diary at the end of every day, and to complete a Worry Episode Log whenever you notice an episode of worry occurring.[5]. We will be using the information that you collect on these forms in our next session. [See Chapter 4, p. 73, for ways to address noncompliance with filling out these forms.]

Figure 3.2 shows a Worry Episode Log completed by Richard for another episode.

ASSESSING PROBLEMATIC PATTERNS IN PAST AND CURRENT RELATIONSHIPS

Poor-quality interpersonal relationships are an important complicating factor in treatment. If other assessments so far have indicated significant relationship problems, the further assessment of these is helpful.

There are several methods for assessing interpersonal difficulties. These include administering the Inventory of Interpersonal Problems Circumplex Scales (IIP-C), looking for patterns across relationships in the client's life, conducting an in-depth exploration of one important relationship, and using the therapist's own emotional experience with the client to identify problematic interpersonal behaviors. All of these types of assessment can be included as part of the initial assessment. The last type of assessment can also be conducted throughout the course of treatment.

The IIP-C is a self-report measure that was developed by Alden, Wiggins, and Pincus (1990). This instrument has eight scales (Domineering/Controlling, Vindictive/Self-Centered, Cold/Distant, Socially Inhibited, Nonassertive, Overly Accommodating, Self-Sacrificing, and Intrusive/Needy) for assessing interpersonal problems. The IIP-C has strong test–retest reliability (total r =.98; average subscale r =.81) and good alpha (.72–.85) coefficients. On this instrument, individuals with GAD report more interpersonal distress and rigidity than do nonanxious controls. Cluster analyses cited by Borkovec, Alcaine, and Behar (2004) indicated interpersonal styles of being overly nurturing and intrusive (62.1% of clients with GAD). Cold and vindictive, and socially avoidant and nonassertive interpersonal styles were indicated by smaller clusters.

In order for the therapist to assess interpersonal problems, the therapist may ask the client about relationships in his or her life. The inquiry should include familial and intimate relation-

---

[5]If worry is pervasive, the therapist should instruct the client to fill out the Worry Episode Log on a scheduled basis (e.g., 10 A.M., 3 P.M., 10 P.M.) or whenever an intensification of worry is noticed.

WORRY EPISODE LOG (FOR ASSESSMENT)

Day/date/time of episode: _Sun. 2/25—10 A.M._

Circle maximum intensity of anxiety during worry episode.

0	1	2	3	4	⑤	6	7	8
None		Mild		Moderate		Severe		Extreme

Circle amount of control over worry episode.

0	1	2	③	4	5	6	7	8
None		Low		Moderate		High		Complete

Other emotions (e.g., anger, sadness, hurt . . . with intensity ratings): _Annoyed—4_

Worry triggers (internal and/or external): What started the worry? _Seeing my briefcase_

Mind: What is happening in your mind? (Rate how convincing on 0–8 scale: _5_)

Images: _Standing in front of the judge and being told my arguments are irrelevant._

Thoughts, assumptions, beliefs (about self, others, situation, function of worry): _I can't do this. Their_ _expectations of me are too high. I could lose my job. I have to keep going over this to make sure_ _I didn't make any mistakes._

Body: How is your body responding physically? _Muscle tension, restless, tightness in my chest._

Actions/behaviors: What do you do (or not do)? _I'm going in to work to go over the case and_ _my arguments._

How long was the worry episode? _260 min._

FIGURE 3.2. Richard's Worry Episode Log (for Assessment).

ships, as well as important friendships. The therapist should focus the client on providing information about the emotional aspects of those relationships (e.g., "How do/did you feel in relation to [identified person]?" or "Tell me about your experience in this relationship. What is/was it like?"), as opposed to gathering information about the other person or obtaining abstract analyses of issues in those relationships. Clients tend either to express denial of blame or to blame others for problems in relationships. Focusing the clients on expressing their emotional experiences and reporting their behaviors (e.g. "What did you do when you felt this way?") within relationships can counteract these tendencies. Underlying beliefs about relationships can be identified (see the section on uncovering core beliefs in Chapter 5) when a client reports a series of relationships that appear to be full of unresolved conflict and/or disappointment, or are experienced as emotionally disengaged.

When patterns are apparent, an in-depth exploration of one relationship can reveal specific client behaviors that may be creating or maintaining problematic interactions. To gather this information, the therapist should instruct the client to pick a typical disagreement or argument with a particular person, or to revisit a time when the client experienced strong emotion in relation to that person. The client then should be instructed to give a blow-by-blow account of everything that happened (e.g., "What did he [or she] do or say?", "What did you do or say?", etc.). The client is not to give his or her perspective or interpretation of what happened, but rather to give a detailed description of all events before, during, and after the situation, including all behaviors and statements of each individual. The therapist should inquire about the client's emotions in relation to the other's behavior, and the client's emotions while behaving in relation to the other. Inquiring about the other's behavioral responses to the client is important as well. In addition, the client should be asked what he or she wanted out of the interaction and what he or she feared while the interaction was occurring. The next clinical vignette demonstrates this type of assessment.

THERAPIST: Are there problems in any relationships that are bothering you?

CLIENT: Yes. I have a bad relationship with this one woman at work. I'm worried that I'm going to look bad to my boss if I can't get along with this woman.

THERAPIST: Are the problems that you are having with her similar to those in any other relationship?

CLIENT: Now that you mention it, there's something similar about the problems I'm having with this woman to those that I've had with a couple of other women.

THERAPIST: Did something happen recently with this woman?

CLIENT: Yes. I have to work on a case with her, and I can't stand it. She's impossible to get along with. There's constant tension and nasty comments between us.

THERAPIST: Let's talk about one instance where the interaction has gone badly. Can you think of one?

CLIENT: Sure. Just yesterday we had a bad interaction.

THERAPIST: I want you to give me a blow-by-blow account of the entire interaction. I want to know every detail. I want to know the exact wording of what you each said to each other, all of your behaviors with each other, and any other details that are relevant to the interaction.

CLIENT: OK. I'll give you some background information first. We were assigned to work together on this one case. The case is very complicated, so we have to coordinate our efforts to make sure that we are efficient and not both covering the same issues. We also are supposed to strategize on the case. Yesterday, we were supposed to meet. I've been feeling really irritated with her because she acts like she's my boss. She's constantly trying to direct me.

THERAPIST: OK. So let me hear the exact details of the interaction.

CLIENT: She walks in and sits down at the desk, like she owns the place.

THERAPIST: What do you mean, "like she owns the place"? I want you to give me a description of her behaviors, rather than your interpretation of her behaviors.

CLIENT: OK. When she sits down, she leans way back in the chair so that she's looking down at me. She never smiles and never engages in any small talk. She starts talking about business immediately.

THERAPIST: And what do you do and say when you enter?

CLIENT: I sit down, and I don't say anything.

THERAPIST: And what is your body posture?

CLIENT: I mimic her posture and sit the same way.

THERAPIST: And what exactly does she say to you?

CLIENT: The first thing out of her mouth is "Have you researched the issue we discussed last time?" I say sarcastically, "No, I've been twiddling my thumbs since our last meeting." Then she says, "Don't take that attitude with me. Just tell me what you've done." I say, "I did what we discussed. What did you do—anything worthwhile?" She then says, "I did what we discussed." Then we sit in silence for about 2 minutes, glaring at each other. She finally breaks the silence and tells me to look up a certain issue for our next meeting, and tells me the issue she's going to research. I say, "Fine," and we both leave.

THERAPIST: Looking back at this interaction, what were you feeling when you first came into the room?

CLIENT: I was feeling really tense.

THERAPIST: What did you want in this interaction with her?

CLIENT: I wanted her to treat me with respect, like an equal.

THERAPIST: Were you afraid of anything in relation to her?

CLIENT: I was afraid she wasn't going to treat me that way. I was afraid we were going to end up in a fight and not be able to work together effectively.

From this reported interaction, the therapist notes Richard's contributions to the negative interaction. His behaviors and statements are either overly passive or aggressive. He avoids opening the interaction with pleasantries. He sits and speaks in an aggressive manner. He avoids asserting what he wants to work on in the case. He appears to be unaware of how his behaviors are affecting the emotional tone of the relationship and preventing him from getting what he wants from the interaction. The therapist concludes from this information that interpersonal effectiveness techniques may need to be part of Richard's treatment.

The therapist's emotional responses in relation to the client can also be used to identify problematic interpersonal behaviors to target for treatment. One method is for the therapist temporarily to examine the therapy relationship as if it were a friendship, and to imagine experiencing the emotional effects of the client's behavior on the relationship from this perspective (e.g., "If [client] were my friend, how would I feel about this behavior?"). Another method is for the therapist to observe his or her own emotional reactions to the client within the therapeutic relationship, to notice client behaviors that are used to avoid or indirectly communicate negative emotions and/or needs in relation to therapy or the therapist (e.g., changing topics, appearing confused, late arrivals, disagreeing with goals or tasks, sarcastic statements, overcompliance, self-justifying/self-aggrandizing remarks).

ASSESSING PLEASURABLE ACTIVITY

Deficits in pleasurable activity can compound difficulties with controlling worry because alternate foci for attention and/or activity may be insufficient. A form called the Pleasurable Activity Log can be used to gather information on the amount of pleasurable activity within the client's daily life. During the assessment phase (usually between Sessions 1 and 2), the client is instructed to record all pleasurable activities during the week on the Pleasurable Activity Log. (Richard's completed form from assessment is shown in Figure 3.3. A blank copy of the form, suitable for reproduction, appears in Chapter 7 as Handout 7.2.) The following information is to be included on this form. The date, type, and duration of activity are recorded. A subjective rating of the intensity of pleasure experienced during the activity is made. The rating is an average of the degree of pleasure over the entire time spent in the activity. The rating is based on a scale from 0 (representing no pleasure) to 8 (representing extreme pleasure). Comments related to positive and/or negative experiences during the activity (e.g., trouble concentrating, worry, feeling relaxed, etc.) are to be included.

TAILORING TREATMENT TO FIT THE INDIVIDUAL CLIENT

Once the diagnostic assessment is complete, the therapist can begin to tailor a treatment plan for the individual client. The development of such a treatment plan requires careful consideration of the following. First, problematic symptoms must be identified for treatment. Once symptoms are identified, treatment goals are set, and specific techniques are selected for accomplishing those

PLEASURABLE ACTIVITY LOG

Intensity of pleasure								
0	1	2	3	4	5	6	7	8
None		Low		Moderate		High		Extreme

Date	Activity	Duration	Rating	Comments
2/24	Out to eat w/wife	120 min.	4	Partly distracted by work

FIGURE 3.3. Richard's Pleasurable Activity Log.

goals. Next, the therapist must consider the role of medication in treatment. Finally, the length of treatment can be estimated.

The client's symptom profile is established by identifying the frequency, duration, and intensity of worry, and the specific stimulus triggers and cognitive, behavioral, and physiological components that contribute to problematic anxiety and worry. Factors that may complicate treatment should be identified as well, and further assessed if necessary. These factors (see Chapter 1) include coexisting diagnoses, nonresponse to past treatment, and poor-quality interpersonal relationships. The initial diagnostic interview and patient self-report assessment tools are used to identify these factors. Richard provides an example of a relatively straightforward case of GAD. His symptoms are indicative of GAD without concurrent diagnoses. Although there is evidence of interpersonal problems, these problems appear to be related to GAD and not to an underlying personality disorder.

Identifying Symptoms for Change

Using information from all of the assessments described above, the therapist identifies targets for change. In Richard's case, there is no history of previous treatment. Richard's interview and his completed forms (see Figures 3.1, 3.2, and 3.3) indicate that Richard's worry is excessive and activated by a wide variety of stimuli (e.g., his briefcase, the word "work," etc.). Many cognitive distortions occur during his episodes of worry (overestimation of vulnerability/risk/harm, underestimation of ability to cope, etc.). Maladaptive beliefs about the process of worry also emerge, such as "Worry keeps me more focused." With his perceived threats, Richard's problem orientation is poor. This can be seen in his anxious drive to the therapy session, where he exhibited nondifferentiation of major from minor elements of a problem. Specifically, the problem was to secure treatment. The minor element of arriving late to a single therapeutic appointment eclipsed the more major element of driving safely to keep from injuring himself and others on the way to the appointment. Numerous symptoms of excess physiological arousal are present (muscle tension, restlessness, etc.). Richard's anxiety-related behaviors and problem coping include excess checking (e.g., excessively checking time when late), overprotection (e.g., prematurely leaving playground with children), and avoidance behaviors (e.g., procrastination about starting treatment and avoiding pleasurable activities). Problematic interpersonal patterns are evident in Richard's overly passive or aggressive behaviors with others. Pleasurable activity is almost nonexistent in his life at pretreatment.

Setting Treatment Goals and Selecting Techniques

Once symptoms and potential complicating factors are identified, specific treatment goals can be set. With respect to GAD, specific goals are set for reducing the frequency, duration, and intensity of worry. Specific techniques are selected to bring about changes in the cognitive, physiological, and behavioral components, and to reduce the specific triggers to problematic worry. These techniques target each type of problematic symptom. When coexisting diagnoses are present, the treatment plan will need to interweave techniques for other disorders with those for GAD. If coexisting diagnoses include other anxiety disorders or depressive disorders, the targets for cognitive-behavioral treatment (CBT) techniques can easily be extended to cover these other disorders as well. Interpersonal problems may require the inclusion of techniques related to specific problems, such as social skills training, assertiveness or anger control, or techniques to overcome emotional avoidance.

Table 3.4 summarizes Richard's symptoms to be targeted in treatment, general treatment goals, and specific techniques for change. In Richard's case, the plan would be to utilize standard CBT, with an initial treatment goal of achieving at least 50% reduction in the frequency, intensity, and duration of worry episodes. The initial expectation of the duration of treatment would be 16–20 sessions over the course of 4–6 months. Assertiveness training and other interpersonal effectiveness techniques would be included later in the treatment, when it became quite clear that certain problematic patterns of interpersonal interaction were exacerbating symptoms of GAD.

The reader is referred to Chapter 2 for descriptions of the various techniques available for treating GAD. Chapters 1 and 2 provide important information regarding empirical support for different techniques. Some techniques have been researched extensively, while others have only preliminary support. As such, these chapters should be consulted before selecting specific techniques.

Medication in Treatment

Whether medication becomes part of the treatment depends on the degree to which symptoms interfere with the client's ability to function, on the client's response to treatment, and on the client's (and the therapist's) personal preference. In instances where a client's anxiety levels are

TABLE 3.4. Richard's Initial Treatment Plan

Symptom	Treatment goal	Technique
Cognitive distortions/ maladaptive beliefs	Reduce distortions and alter beliefs	Cognitive restructuring (CR) Psychoeducation Hypothesis testing
Muscle tension/restless/ feeling on edge/ hypervigilance	Reduce arousal	Applied relaxation (AR) Diaphragmatic breathing (DB)
Excess checking/ overprotection/avoidance	Reduce frequency	Response prevention Graded *in vivo* exposure Pleasurable activity scheduling
Internal and external stimuli activating worry	Extinction of worry response to stimuli	Scheduled worry time Worry exposure
Excess worry	Reduce frequency, intensity, duration of worry	Self-control desensitization (S-CD) AR
Poor problem orientation	Improve problem orientation	Improving problem orientation
[Later:] Overly passive– interpersonal behaviors	Increase interpersonal behaviors	Assertiveness training and other interpersonal effectiveness techniques

overwhelming or grossly interfering with functioning, the therapist may recommend medication as an adjunct to treatment. Depending upon the client's response to treatment, the therapist may also recommend medication consultations for the purpose of either increasing or reducing medication usage. Consultations with psychopharmacologists, specifically, are recommended for any medicinal changes in the treatment of GAD. In Richard's case, the treatment would consist of psychological intervention. Medication would be considered later if the response to the psychological intervention was inadequate. Medications prescribed for GAD are covered in Chapter 1.

Table 3.5 provides a summary of Richard's session-by-session treatment plan. Treatment objectives for each session are identified. Appropriate client handouts, homework assignments, and assessment tools are noted. The plan in Table 3.6 provides general guidance for the treatment of Richard's GAD; actual treatment, however, rarely proceeds without modification. The following description provides an overview of the actual course of treatment with Richard.

Richard's pretreatment assessment with the ADIS-IV indicated a primary diagnosis of GAD, with a severity rating of 5. His scores on the four self-report measures discussed earlier were as follows: BAI, 24; BDI-II, 9; PSWQ, 68; and GADQ-IV, 20. The Worry Diary indicated 60% of the day spent in worry and 544 minutes per day spent in worry. In treatment, initial exercises during Session 2 revealed excellent imaging abilities already in place; positive imagery assignments were given directly. Three extra sessions of challenging cognitive distortions were required before this part of the cognitive restructuring (CR) technique was fully mastered. Although Richard had to tolerate a fair amount of anxiety at the beginning of Phase I of applied relaxation (AR), he was able to master this technique within the sessions as planned. Two extra training sessions of worry exposure were required before the effectiveness of this technique could be established. Richard felt that the self-control desensitization (S-CD) technique was too time-consuming for his busy schedule. Since Richard showed a good treatment response with several other techniques by Session 8, the number of S-CD practices was dropped to once a week after the second week of practice, and completely eliminated by Session 11.

Richard's midtreatment scores on the self-report measures were as follows: BAI, 14 (down from 24); BDI-II, 8 (down from 9); PSWQ, 55 (down from 68); and GADQ-IV, 13 (down from 20). The Worry Diary indicated 35% of the day spent in worry and 336 minutes per day spent in worry down from 60% and 544 minutes. Richard found CR, worry exposure, AR, scheduled worry time, improving problem orientation, response prevention, and pleasurable activity scheduling to be the most effective techniques for reducing his worry. He practiced these techniques over the remaining course of treatment. To address the problematic patterns of interpersonal interaction that were exacerbating and maintaining some of his symptoms, several supplementary techniques for increasing interpersonal effectiveness (assertiveness training, role plays, reversed role plays, reframing the relationship, and exploring links between current and past patterns) were added to treatment. An additional six sessions were required to cover these techniques. His end-of-treatment scores on the self-report assessments were as follows: BAI, 10 (down from 24); BDI-II, 7 (down from 9); PSWQ, 45 (down from 68); and GADQ-IV, 6 (down from 20). The Worry Diary indicated 23% of the day spent in worry and 92 minutes per day spent in worry, down from the initial 60% and 544 minutes.

TABLE 3.5. Summary of Richard's Session-by-Session Treatment Plan

Session 1 objectives

Present treatment rationale.
Present psychoeducation on anxiety and worry.
Introduce rationale for applied relaxation (AR).
Conduct AR, Phase I (lower-body relaxation exercise).
Homework:
  Review Handout 4.2.
  Self-monitor worry on Handouts 3.1 and 3.2.
  Record pleasurable activities on Handout 7.2.
  Practice AR, Phase I (2x/day); record on Handout 6.1.

Session 2 objectives

Introduce rationale for cognitive restructuring (CR).
Begin CR: Increase awareness of cognitive distortions.
  Give Handout 5.2.
Continue AR, Phase I (upper-body relaxation exercise).
Introduce diaphragmatic breathing (DB).
Introduce positive imagery.
Homework:
  Self-monitor worry on Handouts 3.1 and 3.2.
  Review Handout 5.2.
  Practice AR, Phase I, and DB; record on Handout 6.1.
  Practice positive imagery (2x/day) and rate on Handout 5.5.

Session 3 objectives

Continue CR: Begin challenging cognitive distortions.
  Give Handouts 5.1 and 5.3.
Continue AR, Phase II (release-only relaxation exercise).
Review DB and positive imagery.
Homework:
  Challenge cognitive distortions with Handout 5.3.
  Practice AR, Phase II, and DB (2x/day); record on Handout 6.1.
  Practice positive imagery (2x/day) and rate on Handout 5.5.
  Self-monitor worry on Handouts 3.1 and 5.5.

Session 4 objectives

Continue CR: Review challenges to cognitive distortions.
Continue AR, Phase II (release-only relaxation exercise).
Review DB and positive imagery.
Homework:
  Challenge cognitive distortions with Handout 5.3.
  Practice AR, Phase II, and DB (2x/day); record on Handout 6.1.
  Practice imagery (2x/day) and rate on Handout 5.5.
  Self-monitor worry on Handouts 3.1 and 5.5.

Session 5 objectives

Continue CR: Introduce developing alternative viewpoints.
Continue AR, Phase III (cue-controlled, AR merged with DB).
Introduce rationale for self-control desensitization (S-CD).
Begin to develop hierarchy for S-CD.

(continued)

TABLE 3.5. *(continued)*

Session 5 objectives *(continued)*

Homework:
   Challenge cognitive distortions with Handout 5.3.
   Practice AR, Phase III (2x/day) and record on Handout 6.1.
   Practice imagery (2x/day) and rate on Handout 5.5.
   Continue to fill in hierarchy items on Handout 6.2.
   Self-monitor worry on Handouts 3.1 and 5.5.

Session 6 objectives

Continue CR: Introduce decatastrophizing.
Review AR, Phase III (cue-controlled).
Review and revise hierarchy.
Conduct S-CD exercise with lowest-level item on hierarchy.
Introduce improving problem orientation.
Homework:
   Challenge cognitive distortions with Handout 5.3.
   Practice AR, Phase III (2x/day) and record on Handout 6.1.
   Repeat S-CD exercise 3x/week.
   Self-monitor worry on Handouts 3.1 and 5.5.

Session 7 objectives

Continue CR: Introduce developing rational responses.
Continue AR, Phase IV (differential relaxation).
Conduct S-CD exercise with low-level item on hierarchy.
Introduce rationale for treating behavioral responses.
Continue improving problem orientation.
Homework:
   Develop rational responses with Handout 5.4.
   Practice AR, Phase IV (2x/day) and record on Handout 6.1.
   Repeat S-CD exercise 3x/week.
   Self-monitor worry on Handouts 3.1 and 5.5.

Session 8 objectives

Conduct S-CD exercise with moderate-level item on hierarchy.
Continue AR, Phase IV (differential relaxation).
Introduce response prevention.
Identify pleasurable activities.
Continue improving problem orientation.
Homework:
   Develop rational responses with Handout 5.4.
   Practice AR, Phase IV (2x/day) and record on Handout 6.1.
   Repeat S-CD exercise 3x/week.
   Identify pleasurable activities.
   Self-monitor worry on Handouts 3.1 and 5.5.

Session 9 objectives

Conduct S-CD exercise with moderate-level item on hierarchy.
Introduce hypothesis testing.
Introduce *in vivo* exposure.
Continue AR, Phase IV (differential relaxation).

(continued)

TABLE 3.5. *(continued)*

<u>Session 9 objectives</u> *(continued)*

Homework:
  Repeat S-CD exercise 3x/week.
  Assign hypothesis-testing experiment and pleasurable activity.
  Develop rational responses with Handout 5.4.
  Practice AR, Phase IV (2x/day) and record on Handout 6.1.
  Self-monitor worry on Handouts 3.1 and 5.5.

<u>Session 10 objectives</u>

Introduce scheduled worry time.
Introduce worry exposure.
Conduct in-session worry exposure.
Continue AR, Phase IV (differential relaxation).
Homework:
  Assign worry exposure and record on Handout 5.6.
  Assign scheduled worry time exercises.
  Practice S-CD and AR, Phase IV.
  Schedule pleasurable activities and record on Handout 7.2.
  Fill out the BAI, BDI-II, PSWQ, GADQ-IV, Worry Diary.
  Self-monitor worry on Handouts 3.1 and 5.5.

<u>Session 11 objectives</u>

  Collect midtreatment self-report assessments: BAI, BDI-II, PSWQ, GADQ-IV, Worry Diary.
Review results of midtreatment self-report assessments.
Review effectiveness of specific techniques.
Begin client-generated homework assignments with effective techniques.

<u>Sessions 12–15 objectives</u>

Continue with client-generated homework assignments.

<u>Session 16 objectives</u>

  Collect and review end-of-treatment self-report assessments: BAI, BDI-II, PSWQ, GADQ-IV, Worry Diary.
Prepare client to continue treatment in a self-directed manner:
  Review effective techniques.
  Discuss maintenance and generalization of treatment gains.
  Cover relapse prevention.

<u>Sessions 17–20 objectives</u>

Sessions are reserved for booster sessions, as needed.

CHAPTER FOUR

Socialization to Treatment

Before treatment begins, the client must be familiarized with the fundamentals of treatment. Several important topics should be covered. The therapist provides the client with general information about anxiety and worry, presents the model of worry used in treatment, explains the cognitive-behavioral therapy (CBT) of GAD, and then gives the rationale for utilizing various CBT techniques to monitor and reduce anxiety and worry. All of these topics are discussed with specific reference to the client's individual case. This chapter discusses how to present this information to clients. Potential problems that might arise with individual cases during the socialization process are presented in the last section of this chapter.

GENERAL INFORMATION ABOUT ANXIETY AND WORRY

It is important to provide the client with general information about anxiety and worry (see Handout 4.1) and to relate this information to treatment. There are two important points to cover. One is the relationship between fear, anxiety, and worry. The other is the automatic nature of the cognitive, physiological, and behavioral processes that arise with appraisals of threat to vital interests. The following vignette demonstrates a brief didactic presentation of some of this information to our sample client, Richard. It is ideal if the therapist can use personal examples from the client to illustrate these points.

"I want to give you some basic information about fear, anxiety, and worry. Fear, anxiety, and/or worry arise whenever you perceive a threat to your vital interests. Fear occurs when you sense a threat as immediate and present. Anxiety and worry occurs when you sense a potential threat. The sense of threat can be triggered by something in the environment, or it can arise from an internal sense of not being in control of what is vital to you.

HANDOUT 4.1. The Worry Process

FEAR, ANXIETY, WORRY, AND GENERALIZED ANXIETY DISORDER

We experience fear, anxiety, and/or worry when we sense a threat. When a threat seems immediate and present, fear is triggered. When we sense a threat in the future, anxiety and worry are triggered. Threats can come from people or things around us, or from inside ourselves when we feel unable to control what is important to us. Fear, anxiety, and worry are a part of normal human experience. They are not good or bad. They have important uses, but they also can get in our way.

Fear, anxiety, and worry can be helpful (adaptive) when our sense of threat is accurate. Fear helps by pushing us into immediate action to fight or flee danger. Anxiety and worry helps us to ready ourselves for protective action in the future. But our sense of threat is not always accurate. Fear, anxiety, and worry can be triggered by mistake. Have you ever been startled and jumped when someone came up behind you unexpectedly? You jumped back a little before you could think. It was automatic. This automatic fear response can happen even when the person behind you turns out to be a friend that poses no real threat. Anxiety and worry can work in the same way. We can react automatically with anxiety and worry when we sense a future threat. If we find out soon that the threat isn't real, there's no big problem. But sometimes we don't find out. Worry itself can get in the way of finding out. This is because worry creates the sense that we are one step ahead of the threat. When the threat does not happen, it is easy to believe that worry helped to prevent the danger. This can happen even when there never was a real threat. When we think worry protects us, we tend to worry more and more. When this happens, worry can stop being useful. It can get in our way and disrupt our lives.

When unhelpful worry becomes a continuing problem, a person may have what is called "generalized anxiety disorder" (GAD). In GAD, the experience of anxiety and worry is too frequent, too intense, and/or lasts too long. There are effective treatments for GAD and we describe them in this handout. The goal of treatment is not to get totally rid of anxiety and worry. The goal is to reduce worry that is unhelpful and that gets in your way. Treatment for GAD works by helping you understand and recognize the worry process in yourself and teaches you how to weaken or stop the process.

UNDERSTANDING THE WORRY PROCESS

The worry process is like stepping on the accelerator and brake pedals of your car both at the same time. In other words, worry both speeds up and slows down the anxiety response all at once. Worry intensifies anxiety by identifying all sorts of potential threat and reduces anxiety by focusing attention on gaining control or avoiding threat. If you are in a situation that contains many realistic potential dangers, this combination is ideal. If not, worry wastes huge amounts of energy and creates unnecessary wear and tear on your system.

To help you understand and recognize the worry process in yourself, we have separated the process into four parts:

- A "trigger," which is anything that sets off the process of worry.
- What is in your mind (thoughts and images).
- What you feel in your body (physical sensations).
- How you act or behave.

(continued)

The diagram at the end of this handout shows how these parts link up. Each part can automatically set off another part of the process. You can learn to recognize each part of the worry process in yourself. When you recognize the parts, you can learn ways to interrupt the process. Let's take a closer look at each part.

Triggers

"Triggers" are anything that can start or trigger the process of worry. These are some examples: you see a clock (trigger) and immediately feel threatened by thoughts of missing deadlines at work; you hear a loud noise (trigger) that startles you and get an image of your car damaged by a hit and run driver. Situations, events, objects, or persons can all serve as triggers; so can internal physical feelings such as pain or discomfort. For example: you are thinking about your daughter who is at the movies with a friend (trigger) and suddenly start worrying that they may be approached by a child molester. You can begin to notice what sets off your worry. If you are worrying now, try to remember: What was the trigger?

What's in Your "Mind"

When worry is triggered, your mind has thoughts and/or images of threat or danger to your vital interests. You may think about how vulnerable you are and how well you can (or can't) cope with the danger. You may throw yourself into mental planning or preparation, trying to prevent or hold off upsetting events. You may notice your mind racing from one threatening thought to the next, as if it were running through a forest of dangerous ideas. You may think you are overwhelmed or helpless and out of control, having difficulty concentrating or thinking (your mind goes blank).

What You Feel in Your "Body"

When worry is triggered, your body is physically primed to act. You may feel muscle tension, restlessness, trembling, twitching, shaking, shallow breathing, heart palpitations and/or tachycardia, dry mouth, difficulty swallowing, cold and/or clammy hands, sweating, hot flashes or chills, or the urge to urinate frequently. If this state of readiness goes on for a long period of time, you may experience aches, soreness, nausea, diarrhea, or constipation. You may notice anyone or combination of these bodily sensations.

What You Do in "Action/Behavior"

The bodily sensations are preparing you to act, either by fleeing, fighting, or freezing in the face of danger. Worried people act in ways that can be seen as "flight," "fight," or "freeze" behaviors.

- Flight behaviors can include procrastination, avoidance, evasion, escape, and reassurance seeking (requests for support, advice, and/or assistance).
- Fight behaviors can include checking things numerous times, overprotection, and reassurance seeking.
- Freeze behaviors can include any behavior that is inhibited (stammered speech or halted behavior).

When you are worried, you may notice that you are having trouble staying on one task, or you may find yourself overdoing a task, or you may be having difficulty doing any task at all. You also may notice that you are frequently asking others for assistance or input.

(continued)

HOW GAD IS TREATED

Treatment for GAD focuses on each part of the worry process: triggers, the mind's response, the body's response, and your actions/behaviors.

Help for the Mind in the Worry Process

We will look at your personal worry triggers and ask how accurately you see them. We will look at the thoughts you have when worried, and whether you believe worry helps or hurts you. We will help you better judge the probability of threats and your ability to cope with them. Techniques that may be used include keeping a Worry Episode Log, recognizing thinking errors, and developing more useful ways of seeing or responding to things that cause worry now.

Some worry can be triggered by upsetting thoughts and images that pop into your head and start the process. In the short term, worry can lessen the distress these images cause. But it does not work well in the long term. What does work to provide long-term relief is a careful schedule of facing the images, letting yourself feel distressed, and learning that the distress goes away on its own. This technique is called "Worry Exposure." It helps unlink worry-triggering thoughts and images from the rest of the worry process.

Another technique, called "positive imagery," teaches you to replace upsetting images with positive ones that help relax you and help you feel competent.

Help for the Body in the Worry Process

Fear and worry lead to feeling tense, being easily startled, and experiencing other uncomfortable physical sensations. To help with these sensations, you will learn different types of relaxation exercises. One trains you how to relax your muscles deeply. The other trains you how to relax with deep diaphragmatic breathing. You will learn how to practice these techniques both with worrisome imagery and in real life. When you have fully mastered the techniques, they can be used whenever you notice the start of nonadaptive worry.

Help for What You Do: Fight and Flight Behaviors

Behaviors like overchecking, overprotection, and reassurance seeking can be ways to try to "fight" a threat. Behaviors like procrastination, avoidance, evasion, and reassurance seeking, can be ways to "flee" a threat. But when you are mistaken and there is no threat, you don't need to act in these ways. You can learn to change your actions in response to worry with techniques called "response prevention," "craded *in vivo* exposure," and "pleasurable activity scheduling." Response prevention will help you reduce unnecessary fight or flight behaviors. Graded *in vivo* exposure will help you stop using avoidance behaviors, because you will systematically confront situations you have been avoiding. Pleasurable activity scheduling ensures that you engage in different behaviors that encourage a different focus of attention. Each of these techniques help you collect evidence about whether you really need these fight or flight behaviors.

Help for Managing Your Worry Triggers

You will learn techniques that help you manage your worry triggers and weaken the links that make them start you worrying. These techniques are "scheduled worry time," "worry-free zones," and "mindfulness." With scheduled worry time, you train yourself to limit where and when you will allow yourself to worry.

(continued)

Worry-free zones are similar, except that worry is delayed or put off till later at certain times and places. Over time, the worry-free zones are expanded. With either scheduled worry time or worry-free zones, you learn to let go of worry until a later time. These two techniques interrupt new links and weaken old links between worry and specific triggers. Mindfulness increases your awareness and acceptance of the moment. With mindfulness, you train your mind to stay fully focused on the here-and-now—what you can see, smell, hear, touch, taste, or feel physically from inside. This focus increases your abilities to let go of worry and/or to live with unpleasant physical sensations until they go away on their own.

All of these techniques have been scientifically tested and found to be helpful, but not all of them are useful for everyone. We will look at your worry process and choose the ones that seem most likely to help you feel better.

THE WORRY PROCESS

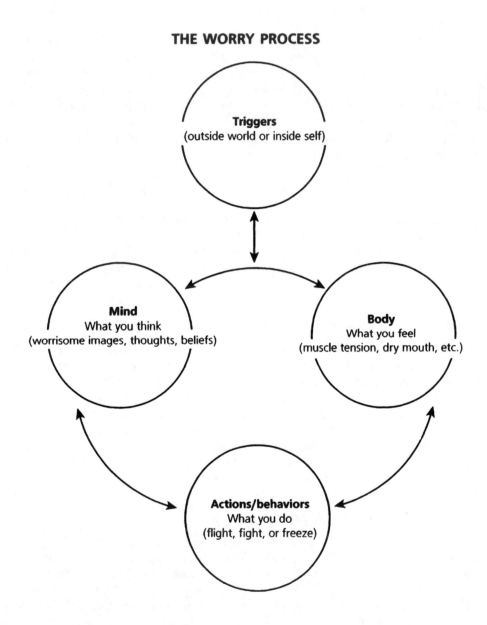

"Fear and anxiety are not bad or good; they are simply emotions that are part of our natural human experience. They can be useful and important, or they can get in your way. Another way to say this is that fear and anxiety can be adaptive or nonadaptive. Treatment is not aimed at eliminating these emotions. The goal is to reduce anxiety and worry that are not useful—that get in your way.

"Let's look at an example to see what happens when fear arises. Let's say you are crossing a street and suddenly notice a car speeding toward you. The car does not begin to brake. Within a split second, three things almost simultaneously occur. Your mind, taking in the sights and sounds of the situation, automatically concludes that the car poses a grave danger to your life and automatically mobilizes specific physiological processes for action (your heart and respiration rates increase, and your muscles tense). Then your body automatically acts in one of three ways, usually described as 'flight,' 'fight,' or 'freeze.' For example, you might run away from the path of the car to avoid the threat. You might scream and wildly wave your arms, fighting to get the driver's attention. You might freeze in your path, which can make it easier for the driver to avoid hitting you. This all occurs very rapidly in a highly coordinated and automatic fashion. If your response to this imminent threat required deliberate thought, physiological mobilization, and action, the car would probably hit you before you had time to act. From an evolutionary perspective, it is clear that the probability of survival is enhanced by the automatic nature of these responses. To recap, fear is an automatic three-part process: (1) Your mind interprets something as a threat; (2) your physical body is readied to act; and (3) you act by fleeing, fighting, or freezing.

"In the speeding-car example, it is obvious that the threat is accurately perceived. Perceptions of immediate threat are not always accurate. You've probably had the experience of someone coming up behind you unnoticed. You may have jumped back startled, maybe even cried out automatically. Perception of potential threat can also be accurate or inaccurate. Problems with worry occur when the perception of potential threat is inaccurate, or when you feel that your ability to cope is insufficient or inadequate. Under such circumstances, worry stops being useful. It starts getting in your way and disrupting your life. Let's now look at an example of problematic worry.

"You're a lawyer, so I want you to imagine yourself in the following situation. You get a negative decision back from the judge. The following cascade of images runs through your mind: You see the client reacting angrily; you imagine the client telling others that you're incompetent; you see your business crumbling, and picture yourself as desperate and unable to find work. In other words, you perceive dire threat to your personal well-being. Your body is tense; your heart is pounding; your breathing is shallow and rapid. In other words, your body physically responds as if your life is in danger. You avoid looking at or thinking any further about the judge's decision, even though you are aware that other problems in this case need to be addressed. Instead, you access your financial records online and start adding up your assets and available cash. You think of ways to cut back on expenditures. You make a gross estimate of how long you could hold out on this money. You feel slightly soothed by this activity, but realize that this is only a temporary solution to the bigger problem. The same perception of threat resurfaces. Your body is aroused again. You begin calling friends and colleagues to see whether there are any new potential referrals. You sound harried and a little desperate for business. Some of those that you have called respond with some new potential business. You go back to your appointment book and begin counting all of your active cases. Again, you are slightly soothed, but you begin to focus on potentially becoming overwhelmed by the number of cases that you may get, in addition to the ones that you already have. You are concerned that your performance will be compromised, and that you may commit malpractice and destroy your business due to overextending yourself. Your heart is pounding fast, and you become very tense once again.

"Your responses would be adaptive, if in fact you were on the verge of a business collapse. It would be adaptive to avoid looking at lost business, and instead to focus on checking, garnering, and attempting to expand resources. In such an instance, your anxiety and worry with their associated problem solving would be useful coping mechanisms. In this instance, however, the threat is not accurately perceived. There is no factual basis to support the frightening images of imminent business collapse. Your mind's interpretation of these images, your physiological mobilization, and your behavioral activities are not helpful. In fact, they get in the way of truly productive behaviors in this situation.

"Now let's look at another way you might react to the same situation. You get a negative decision from a judge. If you interpret the judge's decision as a typical event for all lawyers, you would be free to begin focusing on a strategic approach to the remaining problems in the case. This latter view of events (the judge's decision as part of the everyday events in this business) is a less threatening interpretation. Any worry and associated problem solving could be focused on dealing with actual problems in the case. Rather than focusing on survival concerns, you could focus exclusively on problems related to the task at hand. By staying focused on the task at hand, you would maximize your ability to take control of the situation. The first perception of the event contains a high degree of threat to vital interests, spurring mobilization related to basic survival. Your focus on basic survival necessarily competes with your focus on the task at hand. This dual focus of attention compromises your ability to function efficiently and effectively. This can compound your perceptions of increased loss of control and vulnerability in the situation.

"Worry naturally quells the emotional experience of anxiety, because it spurs and is associated with activities that give us a sense of taking control over events. Worry becomes problematic when it is overused to quell emotion and/or prepare for potential problems. In the example that I just gave, the worry was used to quiet your emotional distress rather than to deal with actual problems in the case. Although the worry provided temporary emotional relief in this situation, the 'reality' of potential threat (the image of imminent business collapse) was left intact and carried the potential for creating bigger problems (drumming up more business than you could handle). As a result, all sorts of unnecessary coping activities occurred. In time, you would have dealt with the concrete problems in the case, and these problems would have been resolved. Your emotional experience, however, would not have helped you to differentiate the worry that spurred productive action from that which interfered. Your emotional experience would have communicated that all of your worry and coping behaviors provided multiple types of relief for all sorts of associated problems. From this example, you can see how easily problematic worry can develop and be maintained."

PRESENTATION OF THE MODEL USED IN TREATMENT

At the end of Handout 4.1 is a visual representation of a model of the worry process that can be used with clients in treatment (see Chapter 2 for further discussion of the model). The clinical vignette continues, demonstrating how this model can be introduced to the client.

THERAPIST: When we sense that our vital interests are threatened, automatic mechanisms in our minds and bodies are activated. Worry specifically occurs when these mechanisms are activated while anticipating the future. Worry can be helpful when it prepares us to cope effectively with a future threat. It is not helpful when it becomes excessive and/or difficult to control. When this occurs, worry interferes with effective and efficient functioning in daily life.

Let's look more carefully at the automatic process associated with worry and how they can be treated. (*Therapist points to diagram at end of Handout 4.1.*) Just as I explained with fear reactions to a speeding car, the experience of anxiety and worry has the same automatic three-part process: "Mind" (cognitive), "Body" (physical), and "Actions/behaviors" (behavioral) (*therapist points to the interconnected circles*). In this diagram, you also see a circle at the top labeled "Worry triggers." Worry triggers are objects or events in your external or internal environment that can start your worrying. External events are concrete objects or situations. These include interpersonal situations. Some examples of external triggers, from what you have told me about your life, are your briefcase and specific behaviors of your boss in relation to you at work. Internal events can be physical sensations or mental images. An example of an internal trigger that you have mentioned is a rapid heartbeat. Worry triggers are anything that has become associated with an interpretation of threat. Can you think of any other triggers?

CLIENT: Sure. Your clock is triggering worry, because it reminds me of how little time I have left for tackling the mound of papers on my desk at work, and I cannot afford to lose my job.

THERAPIST: That's a good example. Now I want you to look at the circle labeled "Mind" (*pointing to circle*). This circle refers to any cognitive event that occurs within our mind during an episode of worry. We refer to this as the "cognitive component" of anxiety. It may be an image, thought, assumption, or belief.

We take for granted that what we think we see, hear, and feel is the same as what occurs in "reality." In actuality, what we know of reality is an interpretation of what we see, hear, and feel. Just as fun-house mirrors can distort our reflections, our minds can distort "reality" by misinterpreting information from our senses. In other words, the "reality" or facts of an event and our interpretation of those facts are not necessarily the same. Sometimes our understanding of the facts bears close resemblance to the "reality," but at other times they may not match at all. For example, a person hears a loud noise outside at night. The person immediately thinks it is a gunshot, but that is an assumption. The "reality" may be that a car backfired. The noise itself is real, but its source is open to interpretation. Cognition also includes daydreams or any other mental imagery. Even without external events, images themselves can trigger worry or make it more intense. When you thought you were running late to our first appointment, you mentioned that you had an image of an angry female therapist on your way here. This image served as both a trigger for worry and a cognitive interpretation of threat. Can you think of any other examples?

CLIENT: (*Pause*) . . . Let's see. This is a little harder.

THERAPIST: Think about my clock . . .

CLIENT: OK. Yes. I see what you're saying. I am thinking that your clock is making me worry, because it is reminding me that I don't have enough time to do my work. But, really, your clock is just a clock. The problems that I have with getting my work done have nothing to do with your clock.

THERAPIST: Right. What are some of the thoughts going through your mind as you are sitting here?

CLIENT: Oh, God (*sighs*). I'm thinking that I'm never going to finish the Harrison matter. That's one of my cases at work. I have so many other matters at work. I really need to get back to work. I can't afford to lose my job.

THERAPIST: So you're having thoughts that you need to keep working to avoid losing your job. Taking time out for therapy is preventing you from getting back to your work.

CLIENT: Yes, and if I lose my job, how would I pay the mortgage and feed my family? What if I couldn't find another job? It took me a long time to get this one.

THERAPIST: So you're thinking ahead to the problems you might face in finding another job. What do you think is the actual probability that you are going to lose your job because you are attending this appointment?

CLIENT: Well . . . it could happen.

THERAPIST: What do you think is the actual probability as the result of coming here this one night?

CLIENT: When you put it that way, it's probably close to zero. But if I keep coming, it could take up more and more time.

THERAPIST: If you continue to put in 11-hour days before coming to this appointment, how likely is it that you will lose your job if you come here after work?

CLIENT: OK, I see your point. It's not likely that I'll get fired simply because I'm taking time for this.

THERAPIST: Right. You just recognized an exaggerated perception of threat, which is generating a whole host of unnecessary responses.

Part of the cognitive component also refers to beliefs—for example, positive and negative beliefs about worry, and beliefs about your ability to solve problems. People who worry too much may also believe they have a general vulnerability to negative outcomes. They may believe that certainty is essential for predicting or controlling events (environmental or social) that are vital. Here are some examples of these beliefs: "Worry lets me stay in control of what happens," "Terrible things are just around the corner," and "I have to plan for every possible contingency. If not, the one that I don't plan will trip me up." Can you think of any beliefs that you have about worry or problem solving?

CLIENT: I'm not sure.

THERAPIST: Beliefs can be hard to recognize because we experience them as simple truths that are beyond question. Let me ask you this: What if you stopped worrying about your work and stopped overworking? What would that mean?

CLIENT: I'd lose control of my cases. My clients would find another lawyer.

THERAPIST: And what would that mean?

CLIENT: That I'm incompetent, a failure, and a loser.

THERAPIST: It sounds like you believe that worry and overworking keep you in control of your cases and your clients, and make you competent and successful.

CLIENT: Yes.

THERAPIST: Is that actually true? You can actually control your cases and your clients by worrying and overworking?

CLIENT: (Pause) . . . Well, when you put it that way . . . no. I can't control my cases or my clients by worrying and overworking. My cases are my cases. Some cases are strong, and some are weak. I can only do my best with each case.

THERAPIST: And what about controlling your clients?

CLIENT: I can't do that, either. My clients will either be satisfied or dissatisfied with the results. I can't control how they react to the outcome.

THERAPIST: So do worry and overwork make you competent and successful?

CLIENT: Actually, it's being disciplined and staying focused on the main issues in a case that increase my chances of being successful. I'm less efficient when I overwork my cases.

THERAPIST: You just recognized a couple of errant underlying beliefs about worry and your competency. These beliefs have been supporting the process of worry.

The cognitive component also refers to the mental strategies you use to cope with the threat. There are two main strategies: avoidance and confrontation. Cognitive avoidance is when you try to turn attention away from something that is emotionally disturbing. Recent thinking is that worry itself may be a method to cognitively avoid something that is emotionally disturbing. An example of cognitive avoidance would be if someone said, "Stop discussing 9/11; I don't want it on my mind." Cognitive confrontation refers to active mental planning and preparation for various threat scenarios. Can you think of any of your own examples of cognitive avoidance or cognitive confrontation?

CLIENT: Oh, man, I'm always thinking of every which way to deal with all sorts of possible problems. I think being a lawyer may make this worse.

THERAPIST: Well, you may have found a profession where cognitive confrontation can be an asset. Is it ever overused?

CLIENT: Definitely. I go way overboard.

THERAPIST: Let's look now at the circle labeled "Body" (*pointing to the matching circle on the diagram*). This refers to physiological responses associated with worry. We call this the "physiological component" of anxiety. When you are worried, you may notice sensations of physiological mobilization, such as muscle tension, restlessness, trembling, twitching, shaking, shallow breathing, palpitations and/or tachycardia, dry mouth, difficulty swallowing, cold and/or clammy hands, sweating, hot flashes or chills, and frequent urination. This physical mobilization has the purpose of supporting any activity that maximizes survival. If your body remains mobilized over a long period of time, you may notice nausea; diarrhea and/or constipation; and muscle aches, spasms, or pain. This physiological mobilization is nothing other than increased activity in the sympathetic division and reduced flexibility in the parasympathetic division of the autonomic nervous system. What physical sensations have you been experiencing while sitting here?

CLIENT: I'm feeling really tense and restless. Whenever I start to worry, I get this tight feeling in my chest. Lately, I've also been getting dizzy and notice a tingling sensation in my hands and feet. Do you think I could be having a heart attack?

THERAPIST: No. Given your clean bill of health, I don't think you are having a heart attack. The symptoms you are mentioning are characteristic of increased physical arousal. I notice that you sigh and take in deep breaths quite often.

CLIENT: My wife says that, too. I'm not aware when I'm doing this.

THERAPIST: When we are stressed or anxious, all of us have a tendency to take shallow breaths and then large breaths. The tightness in your chest, dizziness, tingling, and sighing may be signs that you are breathing in this way. Muscle tension and restlessness also indicate a high state of arousal. All of these sensations are symptoms of the physiological component of anxiety and worry.

This other circle on the bottom is labeled "Actions/behaviors." During episodes of excessive and difficult-to-control worry, you may perform certain behaviors excessively, or you may simply experience strong urges to act. These behaviors are broadly grouped as "flight" and "fight." Escape, avoidance, and procrastination are flight behaviors. An example of avoidance is never traveling by airplane out of worry over terrorism. Excess preparation, checking, and overprotection are all fight responses. For example, preparation becomes excessive if you spend a full day of work extensively researching a minor matter that could have been completed in a couple of hours. An example of overprotection would be if you prohibited your 10-year old from walking to school with friends in a safe neighborhood. Excess checking would be rereading and editing a term paper until it is virtually without error. Reassurance seeking can be seen as either flight or fight: flight to a protective figure, or fight by checking. For example, going to the doctor repeatedly for common minor ailments would be excessive reassurance seeking.

Earlier in our session, you mentioned that you wanted to leave and go back to work. From your posture, it looks as if you are still experiencing this urge to act.

CLIENT: (*Observes himself sitting at the edge of his chair, as if ready to lunge.*) Yes, I guess I do look that way. (*He sits back in the chair, but appears uncomfortable in this position.*)

THERAPIST: Most often, these urges are acted on. From what you told me in an earlier session, it sounds like one of the main ways that you relieve worry is to work.

CLIENT: Yes. I work myself until I'm exhausted. I fall asleep, get up, and start working myself to exhaustion again. It's the story of my life.

THERAPIST: It sounds pretty unpleasant. Do you ever take out any time for pleasurable activities?

CLIENT: Rarely.

THERAPIST: And is there a cost to this?

CLIENT: Sure. My wife and my kids are not happy with me. And I'm not very happy.

THERAPIST: Overworking appears to be one of the behaviors that we'll need to address in treatment.

When one component of the worry process is activated, other components can be automatically activated by way of association. That is what the arrows between all of these components indicate. Think about this example. You experience a sharp pain in your neck (*pointing to "Worry triggers"*). Instantaneously your mind thinks, "Something's wrong" (*pointing to "Mind"*), and your muscles slightly tense (*pointing to "Body"*). All three components are activated, but that's not necessarily the end of the process. The tensing of muscles slightly increases the pain. Then "cancer" pops into your mind, along with an image of being deathly ill in a hospital bed (*pointing to "Mind"*). This spurs more arousal (*pointing to "Body"*). You go to call the doctor and check your neck in the mirror (*pointing to "Actions/behaviors"*). You feel the pain as you look (*pointing to "Worry triggers"*). You start thinking about your life insurance policy and whether to increase benefits to your survivors (*pointing to "Mind"*), and so on and so forth. . . .

As each component sets off another, the intensity of the worry grows, and the episode lasts longer. To decrease the frequency, intensity, and duration of worry, we are going to use two general treatment strategies. One strategy is to target and alter specific elements in each cognitive, physical, and behavioral component of worry. The other strategy is to weaken the associations between the triggers that activate the anxiety/worry process and each component.

PRESENTATION OF THE TREATMENT RATIONALE AND TECHNIQUES

Clients frequently enter treatment with the conception that excessive and difficult-to-control worry is a fundamental part of their being, particularly when their worry is pervasive and has been chronic for many years. It is important to frame a client's problems with worry as habitual patterns that can be altered with a variety of techniques.

If the client is not familiar with the nature of CBT, the following basic tenets of this type of therapy may need to be covered in the client's orientation to treatment:

1. Treatment is focused primarily on the present; explorations of past experiences only occur if they are related to the presenting problems.
2. The goal of treatment is the alleviation of symptoms.
3. Therapy sessions are structured with this goal at the forefront.
4. The relationship between therapist and client is collaborative; they work together as a team toward positive change.

Individuals with GAD appraise inordinate amounts of information as indicating potential threat to vital interests. Although the causes for this overinclusive appraisal of threat are not yet clear, many techniques can be used to alter these appraisals and interrupt associated processes. Any time information is appraised as a threat to vital interests, there is an automatic physiological response. This physiological response keeps a person's mind and body in a state of readiness for any necessary action that may be required to obtain or sustain the fundamentals of life. Plans for action are sometimes executed, either automatically or deliberately. Many appraisals and associated processes occurring during episodes of worry are automatic (meaning that they are not conscious and/or deliberate) and are self-sustaining. The goal of treatment is to reduce the intensity, frequency, and duration of excessive worry by interrupting the automatic nature of the cognitive, physiological, and behavioral processes that contribute to the activation or maintenance of this state of readiness.

Treatment attempts to make changes in, and between, all components of worry. Of the numerous techniques available for reducing worry, some primarily target only one component, while others target multiple components. An overview of the techniques is provided in Chapter 2, and extensive discussions of the applications of specific techniques appear in Chapters 5–8. The following vignette demonstrates how the techniques can be introduced to the client in our sample case, Richard. Again, this didactic presentation ideally incorporates examples from the client's experience, as we've done below with Richard.

"To bring about changes in the cognitive component [pointing to the 'Mind' circle in the Handout 4.1 diagram], you will learn 'cognitive restructuring' exercises. These exercises will show you how to recognize and identify any distortions in your perceptions, and then will help you develop more useful ways of seeing and responding to events that start or intensify your worry now. Some exercises will help you become a better judge of probable versus improbable threats, and others will help you assess realistically how well you can cope with the probable threats. For example, earlier in our session, you said that you felt the threat of losing your job because you were coming to therapy. After you answered a series of questions about the specifics of your situation, you recognized that this threat was highly improbable. You will be learning to apply similar questions to your own thoughts to expose these types of distortions. Part of this treatment is that both of us adopt a scientific attitude about the accuracy of your images, thoughts, assumptions, and beliefs. This means that perceptions or interpretations of events must be treated as hypotheses or guesses, rather than as established truths about events. Images, thoughts, assumptions, and beliefs are evaluated for how well they fit the concrete facts of events. This is in contrast to manipulating, selectively ignoring, or not seeking facts in order to justify or maintain certain perceptions or interpretations of events. Sometimes the recognition that certain interpretations are not factually based is sufficient to enable you to let go of worry, but other times you may need to collect facts to validate an alternative interpretation. In line with this, you will learn how to create experiments to test your hypotheses regarding outcomes with different responses to specific situations. Hypothesis testing allows you to collect concrete evidence regarding feared consequences when your coping activities are altered.

"Sometimes emotionally disturbing or catastrophic images can trigger worry. Although worry can be a way to minimize the immediate emotional distress evoked by such images, it does not work well in the long term. A technique called 'worry exposure' helps you to obtain long-term relief from such images through purposeful and repeated exposures to them. Through the course of these exposures, you will find that the disturbing images are becoming less 'worrisome.' For example, when we see a horrific image for the first time on the news, it is initially emotionally upsetting—but after repeated replays, our emotional reaction diminishes. We eventually habituate to the image.

"We will also be experimenting with a technique called 'positive imagery.' With this technique, you can learn to replace upsetting and disturbing images with positive ones that evoke relaxation or a feeling of competence.

"You can't be tense and relaxed at the same time, so you will be learning different types of relaxation exercises to counter excess physical arousal [pointing to the circle labeled 'Body']. Some of the symptoms of this arousal that you mentioned earlier in our session are muscle tension and increased heart and respiration rates. One of these exercises trains you how to purposefully bring about deep muscular relaxation. The other trains you how to relax yourself with deep diaphragmatic breathing. When these techniques are fully mastered, they can be used whenever you notice the onset of nonadaptive worry. You will learn how to practice applying these techniques in imagery and in real life.

"You will learn to alter your behavioral responses [pointing to the 'Actions/behaviors' circle] with techniques called 'response prevention,' 'graded *in vivo* exposure,' and 'pleasurable activity scheduling.' Response prevention will help you reduce unnecessary coping behaviors. With this technique, you learn how to systematically eliminate unnecessary coping behaviors through structured exercises. As an example of response prevention, you are practicing this technique right now by not leaving my office and staying for the therapy session. Graded *in vivo* exposure helps eliminate avoidance behaviors by having you systematically confront situations that have been avoided. Pleasurable activity scheduling ensures that you execute alternative behaviors that encourage an alternative focus of attention. Each of the behavioral techniques allows you to collect concrete evidence regarding feared consequences when specific behaviors are altered.

"You also will be learning techniques to help you regulate stimuli that evoke the worry process [pointing to the 'Worry triggers' circle], and to weaken the worry response to these stimuli. These techniques are called 'scheduled worry time,' 'worry-free zones,' and 'mindfulness.' Scheduled worry time helps you to regain control over the stimuli that evoke worry, as well as over the automatic response of worry to these stimuli. With this technique, you train yourself to place tight restrictions on where and when you permit yourself to worry. Worry-free zones are similar, except that worry is delayed or postponed during certain times and locations. Over time, the worry-free zones is expanded. These two techniques interrupt new, and weaken old, associations of worry with specific stimuli. With mindfulness, you train your mind to stay fully focused on the present. Mindfulness increases your awareness and acceptance of the moment. For example, these techniques could be used right now to regulate the worry that has been triggered by my clock. With either scheduled worry time or worry-free zones, you let go of your worry until a later time. And with mindfulness, you purposefully turn your attention to stimuli within the here-and-now (e.g., sights, sounds, tactile and internal sensations, etc., of this very moment). The focus of attention on the here-and-now increases your abilities to let go of worry and/or tolerate unpleasant physiological sensations."

PROBLEMATIC CLIENT RESPONSES IN THE SOCIALIZATION TO TREATMENT

The following discussion addresses a number of issues that may arise in the initial phase of treatment.

The Client Does Not Feel That the Rationale Applies to Him or Her

Once the therapist has presented the rationale for treatment, the client may express the belief that it does not apply to his or her case. It is important for the therapist to accept that this may be a legitimate concern. The therapist should acknowledge that this type of therapy brings about significant improvement in about 50%–60% of cases, but that our current state of knowledge does not allow us to determine definitively who will have a positive response. The therapist can suggest that the client try experimenting with the treatment to see whether benefits result. However, it is important to note that most patients get some benefit from the treatment.

The Client Strongly Believes That the Problem Is Strictly Biological in Nature

Despite the explanation of the treatment rationale, the client may remain convinced that his or her problem is purely biological in origin. Here, the therapist can acknowledge that research has not allowed us to determine definitively the degree to which generalized anxiety problems are due to nature versus nurture. Certainly one's inherited temperament plays a role in anxiety. Nevertheless, research has demonstrated that generalized anxiety can be significantly reduced through CBT interventions. Again, the therapist can suggest that the client adopt a scientific attitude toward the treatment to determine whether he or she can benefit from this type of psychological intervention, even if the problem is regarded as primarily biological in nature.

The Client Has Difficulty Identifying Automatic Processes

When a client has trouble identifying automatic processes, the therapist can try presenting hypothetical situations with which the client may identify. Typical automatic processes of an individual with GAD should be included in the example. Sometimes this will be sufficient to spur recognition of such processes. In addition, the therapist can acknowledge differences in awareness of these processes. When processes are extremely automatic, clients simply have to pay extra attention to catch what occurs during episodes of worry. The client can be assured that he or she will get better and better at catching these processes with repeated practice.

Record Keeping Is Inadequate

When records have not been completed or lack useful information, it is important for the therapist and client to work together to determine the exact problem with successful completion. A problem-solving approach is usually the most effective way to remedy the situation. There are numerous possibilities.

One problem may be simply that the client has an inadequate understanding of the important relationship between these records and progress in therapy. The client may believe that his or her worries are "real" and may not understand the reasons why they should be recorded. In this case, reviewing and exploring the client's understanding of the purpose of treatment and the relationship of the records to treatment may prove useful.

Another problem may be that the client has low motivation to make any changes. Perhaps a mate pushed the client to start therapy, but the client is not sufficiently distressed by the symptoms to initiate changes. A cost–benefit analysis may be useful in this instance to help the client determine whether or not to be in therapy at this point in time. The analysis is conducted by dividing a sheet of paper into four sections and labeling each section as follows: "Advantages of treatment," "Disadvantages of treatment," "Advantages of no treatment," and "Disadvantages of no treatment." The client then generates and lists as many short- and long-term advantages and disadvantages as possible for each option. Being able to see the number of items in each section of the page often convinces the client of the importance of following through with treatment.

A third problem may be related to a time management skill deficit in the client. In this instance, part of the session may need to be spent in training the client how to manage his or her time better (see Chapter 8 for a full description of time management training).

A fourth problem may be that the client has weak self-discipline. In this instance, the therapist can implement strategies that provide some structure for the client, such as asking the client to commit to leaving a message for the therapist every day after the assignments have been completed.

Even when records have not been kept, the therapist can use several techniques to capture necessary information—such as asking the client to reexperience events in imagination, to role-play situations, or to reexamine events as if the client were watching a movie frame by frame. The following clinical vignette demonstrates the therapist helping the client reexperience an event in imagination for the assessment version of the Worry Episode Log.

THERAPIST: Great! You've brought in a number of forms. This is going to be very helpful. Before I look at them, do you want to call my attention to anything in particular?

CLIENT: Yes. On Tuesday, I had a really bad day, but I couldn't identify many thoughts.

THERAPIST: OK. Let's start with that one. . . . You have down here that you were at work, and you rated your anxiety at 7.

CLIENT: Yes. I was really anxious that day.

THERAPIST: You've got this down under "Thoughts, assumptions, beliefs": "I'm so anxious. I can't focus. I'm not going to get this assignment done."

CLIENT: Yes. That was the only thought I noticed, and it kept going through my head. I was anxious about getting that assignment done, which I think was normal, but my anxiety was so high I was having trouble concentrating. I couldn't sit still at my desk. It was ridiculous.

THERAPIST: Sometimes it is difficult to identify automatic processes, particularly when you're in a situation where you don't have a lot of time to reflect on what's going through your mind. I'm going to show you a technique that can help. With this technique, you recall the situation in your imagination. Do you want to try it?

CLIENT: OK.

THERAPIST: Can you remember where you were and what was happening before you noticed an increase in your anxiety?

CLIENT: Not really. I was at my desk all day.

THERAPIST: What were some of the events that occurred that day?

CLIENT: (Pause) . . . At one point, my boss came in to ask me about a memo. Yeah, that happened before I started feeling really anxious.

THERAPIST: Good. Let's focus on the time right before your boss walks into your office. I want you to close your eyes. . . . Now, try to picture your office. . . . Let yourself feel as if you are actually there. . . . Picture the inside of your office . . . the color of the walls . . . the lighting . . . picture your desk . . . feel yourself sitting at your desk . . . in your chair . . . hear the sounds in the office . . . the smells . . . recall what it feels like to be there. . . . Now tell me what's happening.

CLIENT: I'm sitting at my desk. . . . I see piles of papers in front of me. I'm holding my pen and I'm looking at the Grieg matter. . . . I hear my boss walking down the hall toward my office. His footsteps sound deliberate. I feel tense. I think I've done something wrong. . . . He walks into my office. He asks, "Do you have the memo on that issue in the Kelly case?" My mind is racing. My heart is pounding. I'm sweating. I stumble on the words, "I don't have it done." He says, "Get it to me as soon as you can," and leaves abruptly. . . . I'm sitting at my desk, alone in my office. My mind replays the events, but I see him yelling, "You're fired!" I feel panicked and under intense pressure. I'm thinking, "I have to get this done!"

THERAPIST: Good. Let's stop for a moment. You can open your eyes. . . . Now, fill in the form with what you just uncovered.

In the vignette above, it is clear that Richard originally was not fully conscious of some aspects of this episode of worry. He was primarily aware of the sensations of anxiety and of the worry about his productivity as the result of his high level of anxiety. For the therapist who is not experienced in working with such clients, the client's lack of awareness of some of the cognitive processes can lead to confusion about the purpose of the forms. For example, this client's worry about his productivity is reasonable, given his difficulties with concentrating. To target these worries would be fruitless, however, as they make logical sense and are supported by the concrete facts of the situation. In such instances, the therapist and the client should closely and carefully examine all of the external and internal events that immediately preceded the onset of the worry episode. This process often spurs memory of ignored events and various automatic processes that led to later reality-based problems, as in the example above.

The Client Believes That High Levels of Anxiety Are Dangerous

A frequently encountered misconception is that high levels of anxiety are dangerous. The danger may appear as concern that it can cause a heart attack or insanity.

With respect to concerns about heart attacks, clients can be told that the high states of physiological arousal during high levels of anxiety are not dangerous when people are in good physical health. It is normal and natural for arousal to increase substantially when any threat to vital interests is processed. Human bodies, however, also have a built in protective mechanism called the parasympathetic nervous system, which prevents arousal from spiraling upward endlessly or becoming endless. The parasympathetic nervous system, which is responsible for putting the body into a relaxed state, eventually kicks in when arousal gets too high or lasts too long. High arousal increases the chances of a heart attack only if other risk factors are present. A client's physician can confirm this information.

Regarding concerns about insanity, clients can be told that high levels of anxiety do not cause people to become psychotic. Sometimes clients develop this misconception from their awareness that they have difficulties concentrating and/or thinking when they are highly anxious. It is important to tell clients that these difficulties result from their being in a hypervigilant state. When highly aroused during intense episodes of worry, the mind is actively scanning for any sign of potential danger. This is the same type of scanning that would occur if clients were in a situation where their lives were potentially in danger (e.g., alone without a weapon in a jungle where fierce wild animals were known to roam). In such a situation, it would not be adaptive to concentrate deeply or think through complex problems. Rather, rapid shifting of attention and superficial processing of environmental stimuli occur. These types of mental activity are adaptive in such situations and are vital aspects of healthy brain functioning. They are not representative of insanity. These types of mental activity are completely different from the thought disorders associated with psychosis and do not cause psychosis.

Although part of the treatment provides relaxation techniques for modifying arousal, they are not provided because arousal is considered dangerous. In fact, many techniques for anxiety reduction initially require the client to tolerate increased arousal. Tolerating arousal until the parasympathetic nervous system is activated (either naturally or with techniques) is related to achieving long-term reductions in the frequency, intensity, and duration of this arousal.

The Client Has Had a Paradoxical Response to Relaxation

On occasion, there will be a client who resists the idea of relaxation exercises. In such instances, it is important to explore the reasons for resistance. The most challenging reason is that the client has tried relaxation before and had the paradoxical response of increased anxiety when attempting to relax. This response can occur for a variety of reasons. Often there is a meaning associated with the relaxation response that needs to be addressed. The meanings may include that relaxation is too self-indulgent, that it's a waste of time, that it represents a loss of control, or that the sensations may be associated with panic sensations. The next two chapters cover ways to challenge and test these types of interpretations about relaxation.

CHAPTER FIVE

Treating the Cognitive Component

Individuals with GAD are masters at identifying potential threats to their vital interests and can become entrenched in attempts to control potential negative outcomes. These attempts can be cognitive and/or behavioral. This chapter focuses on treating the cognitive component of GAD. The phrase "cognitive component" refers specifically to images, thoughts, assumptions, and beliefs that are related to the process of worry in GAD. These images, thoughts, assumptions, and beliefs may concern specific stimulus events or the process of coping with threat. Several techniques can be used to bring about cognitive change. They include cognitive restructuring (CR), positive imagery, worry exposure, improving problem orientation, cost–benefit analysis of coping, scheduled worry time, and worry-free zones (see Table 5.1). This chapter describes each of these techniques in detail. The treatment techniques for altering the behavioral component of GAD will be discussed in Chapter 7.

COGNITIVE RESTRUCTURING

In CR, the client learns how to recognize and evaluate the validity of his or her interpretations of events, and how to generate and test alternative and possibly more adaptive interpretations. CR is accomplished in four basic steps (see Table 5.2). The first step is to increase awareness of cognitive activity during episodes of worry. The second step is to systematically challenge nonadaptive cognitions. The third step is to generate alternative viewpoints. The fourth is to create and test more adaptive cognitive responses.

TABLE 5.1. Techniques That Target the Cognitive Component of GAD

Psychoeducation	Positive imagery
Cognitive restructuring (CR)	Worry exposure
Worry Episode Log (for Treatment)	Improving problem orientation
Guided discovery	Cost–benefit analysis of coping
Decastrophizing	Cognitive response prevention
Developing alternative viewpoints	Scheduled worry time
Hypothesis testing	Worry-free zones

TABLE 5.2. Steps and Tools for Cognitive Restructuring (CR)

Step 1: Increasing awareness of cognitive activity

Methods
    Worry Episode Log (for Treatment)
    Juxtaposing facts with interpretations of facts
    Education about common distortions in thoughts and assumptions
    Uncovering core beliefs associated with worry

Step 2: Systematically challenging distorted cognition

Methods
    Guided discovery
    Decatastrophizing

Step 3: Generating alternative viewpoints

Methods
    Imagining the event from a third-person perspective
    Switching roles
    Changing the frame
    Taking other emotional perspectives
    Imagining extremes to imagine the middle
    Enlisting the help of others

Step 4: Creating and testing rational responses

Methods
    Rational Response Form
    Hypothesis testing

Step 1: Increasing Awareness of Cognitive Activity

The first step is to heighten the client's awareness of cognitive activity during episodes of worry. Awareness can be increased through several methods. One method is to use the version of the Worry Episode Log that has been designed as a treatment tool (see Handout 5.1). Another method is to juxtapose concrete facts of an event or situation with interpretations of those facts. A third is to educate the client about common distortions in thoughts and assumptions. The fourth is to uncover core beliefs associated with worry. Each method is discussed in the following sections.

Worry Episode Log (for Treatment)

In the assessment phase, episodes of worry are monitored to highlight processes occurring within and between the various components. A modified version of the Worry Episode Log employed in assessment (see Handout 3.2) is used for this purpose during the treatment phase (see Handout 5.1). The treatment version includes a section for recording interventions. In addition to increasing awareness of automatic processes, the modified log facilitates awareness of when and where treatment techniques can be applied; it also increases awareness of the effectiveness of specific interventions. The following clinical vignette demonstrates how to make the transition from using the assessment version to the treatment version.

> "It is important for you to continue monitoring worry throughout treatment. Monitoring helps you to become more and more aware of processes that are occurring on an automatic level. As you observe these processes, it will become easier to recognize where and how you can stop the worry process with the techniques you will be learning.
>
> "Instead of using the version of the Worry Episode Log you used at the beginning, I want you to begin using a version that has been modified for treatment [gives Handout 5.1 to client]. As you can see, this new form includes a section labeled 'Intervention' [points to section]. This new section is used to record what specific techniques are used during an episode and the effectiveness of the applications. This will help us assess the effectiveness of particular techniques in reducing nonadaptive worry."

Juxtaposing Concrete Facts and Interpretations of Facts

Individuals commonly experience their interpretation of an event as the "reality" of that event. This method of juxtaposing facts and interpretations is aimed at increasing the client's awareness of the difference between the concrete perceived facts of an event and the images, thoughts, assumptions, and beliefs evoked by the event. The process begins with selection of a specific incident, usually taken from either the assessment or treatment version of the Worry Episode Log. The therapist first validates the client's anxiety response, given the interpretation of threat. Then the therapist questions the client to draw out all the relevant facts, helping the client distinguish them from images and cognitions. As the facts are reviewed, the therapist checks with the client on whether the worry process was triggered by the facts or the interpretation. The next clinical vignette demonstrates this process. (Again, the client is Richard, the anxious lawyer).

WORRY EPISODE LOG (FOR TREATMENT)

Day/date/time of episode: _____

Circle maximum intensity of anxiety during worry episode.

0	1	2	3	4	5	6	7	8
None		Mild		Moderate		Severe		Extreme

Circle amount of control during worry episode.

0	1	2	3	4	5	6	7	8
None		Low		Moderate		High		Complete

Other emotions (e.g., anger, sadness, hurt . . . with intensity ratings: _____

Worry triggers (internal and/or external): What started the worry? _____

Mind: What is happening in your mind? (Rate how convincing on a 0–8 scale: ___)

    Images: _____

    Thoughts, assumptions, beliefs (about self, others, situation, function of worry): _____

_____

_____

Body: How is your body responding physically? _____

_____

Actions/behaviors: What do you do (or not do)? _____

_____

Interventions: What treatment techniques do you use, and how well do they work? _____

_____

_____

How long was the worry episode? _____

THERAPIST: It says here (*looking at the assessment version of the Worry Episode Log*) that on Sunday, you were at the playground with your daughter. She was climbing on the jungle gym, and she slipped. You rated your anxiety at 6. When this occurred, you noticed the following thoughts, "Oh, my God, she almost fell. She could get seriously hurt. I have to stay on top of everything she's doing." The strength of your belief in those thoughts was 95%. Physical sensation was muscle tension. Your behaviors were to tell her to be more careful, to move closer to where she was playing, and to watch her very closely. You left the playground early.

CLIENT: Yes. Playgrounds make me so anxious.

THERAPIST: I want you to listen to what you just said. You said, "Playgrounds *make* me so anxious." I've stressed the word "make," because people frequently believe that situations make them feel certain ways. I would like to use this event to take you through an exercise. This exercise will help you to differentiate the concrete facts of the situation from your interpretation of that situation. What were the concrete facts in this situation?

CLIENT: My daughter was playing on the equipment, and she slipped.

THERAPIST: When you say she slipped, can you tell me exactly what you saw?

CLIENT: She was climbing on the equipment, and her foot slipped off one of the bars.

THERAPIST: And what was your interpretation of those facts? In other words, what went through your mind when her foot slipped off the bar?

CLIENT: That she almost fell, that she could get seriously hurt on this equipment, and that I have to stay on top of everything she's doing.

THERAPIST: Good. These are the concrete facts of the situation: Your daughter was climbing on the equipment, and one foot slipped off the bar. These are your thoughts about this situation: "She almost fell; she could get seriously hurt; I have to stay on top of everything she's doing." Most people experience the situation and their interpretation of the situation as one and the same. I just asked you to separate the two. What do you notice about your interpretation of the situation?

CLIENT: I was thinking she almost got seriously hurt.

THERAPIST: Right. Your interpretation of the situation contains potential for serious threat to your daughter's well-being [validation of anxiety, given interpretation of threat].

CLIENT: (*Richard looks down, shakes his head, and sighs.*) If she ever suffered a permanent injury, I could never forgive myself.

THERAPIST: What just went through your mind when you hesitated a few moments ago?

CLIENT: I saw her lying on the ground, paralyzed.

THERAPIST: And how are you feeling?

CLIENT: Anxious again.

THERAPIST: I want you to notice that you just experienced a threatening image, even though we and your daughter are nowhere near a playground. The image is not the actual situation; yet you are experiencing distress as if this danger is hovering. Let's take a step back and look again at the concrete facts of the situation. What actually happened when her foot slipped off the bar?

CLIENT: Nothing.

THERAPIST: Nothing? She just stayed in that position?

CLIENT: No. She grabbed on to the bar very tight.

THERAPIST: And?

CLIENT: She didn't fall.

THERAPIST: And?

CLIENT: She kept playing.

THERAPIST: So in the actual situation, she slipped, caught herself, and continued to play. Let's go back to your original interpretation. You had the thoughts, "She almost fell; she could get seriously hurt; I have to stay on top of everything she's doing." Later, in this office, you noticed that you had an image of her lying paralyzed on the ground as you thought back to the situation. How are you interpreting this playground situation?

CLIENT: I see what you're saying. I'm interpreting playing at the playground as a very dangerous endeavor.

THERAPIST: Right. I want you to notice the difference between the concrete facts and your interpretation of these facts. It's not the situation itself that makes you anxious. Your daughter, playing on the equipment in the playground, does not make you anxious. Rather, it is the interpretation of danger and threat in this situation that is affecting how you are feeling.

Identifying Cognitive Distortions

When everything except elements of danger or threat is filtered out of a client's perception of events, the degree of danger is easily overestimated, and the degree of safety is underestimated. Overestimation of danger and underestimation of safety are two major cognitive distortions that occur in the interpretation of events in individuals with GAD. As the perception of risk increases, distortions in the cost–benefit ratio of coping responses also become apparent.

Overestimation of danger and underestimation of safety can be recognized in various specific types of distortions, such as catastrophizing, faulty estimates, gross generalizations, and polarization. Minimization of protective factors may also be evident. Distortions related to coping responses can be recognized in minimizations of coping capabilities and/or unrealistic expectations for outcomes.

A handout listing typical cognitive distortions can be given to the client (see Handout 5.2). Discussing this list with the client, and having the client generate examples from his or her own life, can increase awareness of the distortions. The following adds to the descriptions of each type of distortions in Handout 5.2.

COMMON THINKING ERRORS

Errors in Interpretation

Catastrophizing. The worst possible outcomes of events are predicted. Imagining that basic needs for sustenance, safety, connection, autonomy, self-esteem, or self-expression are threatened. Examples: "I'll get fired," "This could be cancer."

Faulty estimates. An inaccurately high probability of danger is estimated. Example: A car weaves slightly within the lane and the driver in the adjoining lane, tells his passenger, "Did you see that guy? He almost hit us!"

Gross generalizations. The danger perceived in one event is inappropriately generalized to other events. Example: A woman hears on the radio that an accident has occurred on a route her daughter occasionally drives. She worries that it's her daughter in the accident.

Polarization. Aspects of danger associated with a person or situation are perceived in absolute black-or-white terms. For instance, situations are viewed as totally safe or totally dangerous; there is no relative degree of danger. Examples: A woman always worries about being attacked any time she enters an elevator with a stranger.

Minimization of safety factors. Facts that indicate protection or safety are minimized or not attended to. Example: "I would never shake the hand of someone who has AIDS."

Errors Related to Coping

Minimization of coping capability. Expressions of a lack of control or helplessness are not in line with capabilities. Examples: "I couldn't deal with it," "I don't know what I would do."

Unrealistic expectation for outcome. Expectation for outcome is expressed in absolute terms of perfection, certainty or control. Example: "I have to do everything possible to make sure there are no mistakes."

Distortions in Interpretation of Events. Catastrophizing is evident when the individual's thoughts focus exclusively on the worst possible outcomes of events. These outcomes contain threats to the individual's ability to survive or thrive. Any of the basic needs for sustenance, safety, connection, autonomy, self-esteem, or self-expression may be threatened. For example, a man who is having trouble finding time to do his taxes starts to worry that he'll be thrown in jail.

Faulty estimates are evident when the probability of danger is assessed at inaccurately high levels, particularly when the actual probability of danger is ambiguous. For example, a man is golfing on a day with a threat of rain. As he plays, he becomes increasingly worried that he'll get caught in a violent thunderstorm in the middle of the course and be electrocuted.

Gross generalizations are evident when the danger perceived in one event is applied to other events, without any differentiation between events. For example, a woman hears on the radio about a mugging in the parking lot of a mall and worries about getting mugged as she walks out of her apartment.

Polarization is evident when events are perceived in all-or-nothing terms of extreme danger or safety. For example, a woman never feels safe driving, despite the facts that she only drives her Volvo during daylight hours in good weather conditions.

Factors that indicate protection or safety may be minimized or ignored. For example, a woman hears a tree branch hitting the window of her third-story apartment in a well-lit complex, and worries that the noise is caused by someone breaking in.

Emotional justifications can be recognized when emotions are used to justify the validity of perceptions. For example, an anxious person thinks, "There must be something wrong, because I'm feeling so anxious."

In addition to the singular occurrence of a distortion, distortions may occur en masse. Because large numbers of stimuli have past associations with the idea of danger, the potential exists for the idea of danger to activate a cascade of past associations. The hypervigilance that accompanies high arousal facilitates additional associations of new stimuli with ideas of danger. When distortions occur en masse, the individual feels overwhelmingly threatened and is likely to experience a panic attack.

Distortions Related to Coping. Minimization of coping capabilities may be evident in expressions of a lack of control or helplessness that are out of line with the individual's capability. For example, a bright young man (like Richard) imagines being asked to leave his law firm and worries about ending up living out on the street.

Unrealistic expectations for outcomes are expressed in absolute terms for perfection, certainty, and/or control. For example, a person thinks, "I have to make sure nothing bad can happen."

Uncovering Core Beliefs

Burns (1980) developed a technique called "vertical descent" to clarify deeper meanings or more fundamental beliefs. Vasey and Borkovec (1992) utilized this technique to uncover core beliefs associated with worry. The beliefs accessed through this procedure may be about the self, about others in relation to the self, and/or about worry or the problem-solving process.

When implementing this technique, the therapist should prepare the client for the possibility that he or she may experience an intense level of anxiety. This can occur because the client is focusing and maintaining attention on his or her most threatening cognitions. Sometimes the cognitions present as a cascade of frightening thoughts, assumptions, beliefs, and images. In such instances, the client may feel overwhelmed and panicked by the affect that is evoked. When this occurs, the therapist can have the client observe and record each separate thought, assumption, belief, and image within the cascade. This will help to slow down and weaken the strength of the cascade, and it prepares the client for the next step of challenging individual cognitions. The therapist also may choose to immediately subject any emotionally distressing belief to the methods of guided discovery or decatastrophizing (presented later) within the same session to dissipate some of the affect.

To fully access the deeper meanings or beliefs associated with worry, the client is asked to generate a list of current worries. Each individual worry is then subjected to the following types of questions: "What if [restated worry], then what? . . . And if that were to happen, then what? . . . And what would that mean?" To fully access positive and negative beliefs about the purpose of the worry, similar questions are asked: "If you were to stop worrying about [restated worry], what do you think would happen? . . . And if that were to happen, then what? . . . And what would that mean?"

In the identification of beliefs, the therapist can utilize the following general guideposts. Beliefs about the self or others in relation to the self concern perceived abilities to obtain or control basic needs for survival. Beliefs about worry are related to positive and negative valuing of worry.

Basic survival needs of the individual include both physical and psychological needs. Young and Klosko (1993) suggested six core needs that require an adequate level of fulfillment for psychological health: basic safety, connection to others, autonomy, self-esteem, self-expression, and realistic limits. Queries about the deeper meanings of worry can reveal the threads of connection between specific events and core beliefs regarding the fulfillment of these basic survival needs.

Beliefs about the positive and negative value of worry generally follow two themes (Freeston, Rheaume, Letarte, Dugas, & Ladouceur, 1994). The first is that worry helps to find solutions to problems. The second is that worry can prevent or minimize negative outcomes.

Borkovec and Roemer (1995) found that individuals with GAD have a greater tendency to use worry to distract themselves from more emotional topics. The positive value of worry (which is the problem-solving aspect to prevent negative outcomes) may become negative when worry is misapplied simply to avoid emotional distress. As the result of misapplications of worry, metaworry (Wells, 1995, 1999) may develop. Metaworry relates to cognitive confidence (i.e., concerns about cognitive efficiency, including concerns about memory and attention), and to the uncontrollability of worry and corresponding dangers (mental and physical) associated with worry (Davis & Valentiner, 2000).

An example of increasing awareness of beliefs related to the positive and negative value of worry can be seen in a clinical vignette in Chapter 3. As the therapist helped Richard fill out an episode on the assessment version of the Worry Episode Log, she asked, "What do you believe about the process of worry in these types of situations?" Richard's responses included "Worry keeps me focused on what I'm doing" and "My worry makes others more forgiving of my mistakes." Yet in this case, his worry contributed to unsafe and risky driving. The therapist was then able to highlight the negative value of misapplied worry. The next vignette below demonstrates the process of uncovering beliefs related to the fulfillment of specific basic needs. Richard has just listed his current worries as follows:

1. Not able to make a decent living.
2. Getting a life-threatening disease.
3. One of my kids dies.
4. My wife leaves me.

THERAPIST: Let's take the first worry you've listed to explore the deeper meaning of this worry. We are going to subject this worry to a procedure called "systematic catastrophization." We will later challenge these beliefs, but only after we have arrived at an understanding of the deeper meaning of this worry. Are you willing to try this?

CLIENT: Sure.

THERAPIST: Tell me more about this worry.

CLIENT: I feel really anxious when I have this thought. It brings up this image of being out on the street, dirty, hungry, cold, and alone.

THERAPIST: OK. Try to stick with this upsetting image and tell me—so what if you were not able to make a decent living? What then?

CLIENT: People would look down on me. I'd be shunned.

THERAPIST: And if people shunned you, then what?

CLIENT: I'd be all alone. No one would want to be with me.

THERAPIST: And what would this mean?

CLIENT: I'm unworthy of love and attention.

THERAPIST: So deep inside, you believe that making a decent living protects you from being alone. Otherwise, you are unworthy of love and attention. Is that right?

CLIENT: Yes.

THERAPIST: Where did you learn this idea—that your worth and value as a human being depends upon how you perform financially in the eyes of others?

CLIENT: I'm not sure.

THERAPIST: Let's try to trace this back.

This next part of the vignette uses a schema therapy technique (Young, Klosko, & Weishaar, 2003), which has not yet been empirically validated for treatment of GAD. This technique is used here to clarify the origin of Richard's core belief and for getting at the "emotional topic" to which Richard may be misapplying worry. This same technique, also called "focused exploration of the past," can be used for confronting avoidance of emotion in GAD, as discussed further in Chapter 8.

THERAPIST: I don't want you to use your intellectual side to figure this out. I want you to use your emotional side to trace this back. Try to let your mind float. Use your emotional feelings, the feelings in your body, to trace this back. Try to recall when you first had this feeling in your body, the feeling when you have upsetting images like this.

CLIENT: OK. . . . I always had this feeling with my mom and dad, especially my mom. (*Richard appears more upset*)

THERAPIST: (*Pause*) . . . What is it that you are remembering?

CLIENT: Whenever I did my homework with my mom, she would yell if I made any kind of mistake. She paid so much attention to what I did wrong. She was so harsh and critical. I felt like my work had to be flawless to be acceptable. I felt like I had to be perfect for her to accept me and want to be with me.

THERAPIST: And what about your dad?

CLIENT: My mom always criticized him for not making enough money. It seemed like she could only love him if he made a lot of money. . . .

THERAPIST: And what do you remember about him?

CLIENT: He was always working long hours trying to make more money, but he never made enough to please her. He told me over and over how important it was to do well financially to be successful and happy in life.

THERAPIST: Do you notice any similarities between these emotional memories and the problems that you are experiencing now?

CLIENT: Yes. Now I see why I started becoming so afraid of making any mistakes at work. Mistakes mean I won't be accepted. I'll get fired and then rejected by everyone. I believe my performance has to be perfect for my boss to want me, just like my mom.

THERAPIST: You know, Richard, any event that even hints at the possibility of a problem with your performance may trigger this old, erroneous deeper belief and the powerful feelings that are associated with this belief. . . . We'll have to pay close attention to this possibility.

CLIENT: Yes, I think so.

The vignette above reveals how this belief is related to Richard's chronic worry about his performance at work. His mother's unrealistic standards and excessive criticism, and his father's work behaviors, appear to have contributed to the formation of a deeper belief that Richard will be unacceptable and unworthy of love and attention if his work performance falls short of perfection. Any mistake in performance poses an automatic serious threat to his positive self-esteem and connection with others. This idea that developed in relation to his parents' behavior will need to be repeatedly challenged and tested with cognitive and behavioral techniques in his current work and family environments. Although this general set of parental circumstances may be quite common in the development of chronic worry (Stober & Joorman, 2001), a therapist should be vigilant for any basic needs that may have been threatened or difficult to obtain in the course of a client's development.

Step 2: Systematically Challenging Distorted Cognitions

Once the client reliably identifies images, thoughts, assumptions, and beliefs associated with problematic episodes of worry, the client is ready to learn approaches for challenging these cognitions. We present two techniques for this purpose: guided discovery and decastrophizing. These techniques prevent individuals with GAD from cognitively avoiding emotionally distressing topics associated with worry. They make worries concrete. Stober (1998) has highlighted reduced concreteness as an important contributing factor to chronic worry, and Stober and Borkovec (2002) have provided preliminary evidence of the importance of the concretization of worry for reducing excessive worry and increasing the effectiveness of the problem-solving aspect of worry.

Guided Discovery

Aaron Beck (see especially Beck & Emery with Greenberg, 1985) introduced the Socratic method of questioning cognitions as an effective tool for altering cognitions and thereby emotional responses. This method has also been termed "guided discovery." The goal is to guide the client toward determining whether or not there are factual distortions or logical errors in his or her cognitions. The method is a series of questions.

When the therapist recognizes distortions or errors in the client's thinking, it is of utmost importance for the therapist to refrain from simply telling the client that he or she has made particular errors, arguing with the client, or persuading the client to see the situation from the therapist's perspective. Rather, the therapist's role is to help the client determine for him- or herself whether or not a particular perspective is valid and/or accurate. The therapist can encourage the client to see whether he or she can recognize any distortions from the list of cognitive distortions (Handout 5.2). Or the therapist can accept the client's viewpoint as one of many potentially valid perspectives, and then pose questions (see also "Juxtaposing Concrete Facts and Interpretations of Facts," above) that help the client recognize pieces of information that may have been ignored or distorted. The following clinical vignette illustrates this approach with automatic thoughts.

THERAPIST: Is there anything from the week that you want to discuss?

CLIENT: Yes. I was having a lot of anxiety at the beginning of the week about a difficult case at work.

THERAPIST: Do your Worry Episode Logs for Monday, Tuesday, and Wednesday apply?

CLIENT: Yes. It started Monday with this new assignment. I was very excited at first, because the assignment gives me an opportunity to work with a high-profile client. If I do a great job, my career could really take off. But the assignment is in an area where I'm not an expert, and it's a fairly complicated matter.

THERAPIST: Let's try to identify exactly what happened when this feeling of excitement began to turn into anxiety. First, let's go through the thoughts you wrote down on Monday. You wrote, "If I make a mistake, I could look incompetent. I really don't know what I'm doing. I've got to make sure there are no mistakes."

CLIENT: Right.

THERAPIST: You've identified a whole string of automatic thoughts that we can examine. Let's take one thought at a time. The first thought is "If I make a mistake, I could look incompetent." Can you say with certainty that if you make a mistake, you *will* look incompetent?

CLIENT: Well, I'm not an expert on this subject. I'm bound to make a mistake.

THERAPIST: OK. You are not an expert and possibly will make a mistake. Is it true that making a mistake will result in others' viewing you as incompetent?

CLIENT: It depends on the type of mistake. If I make a major mistake, I'll probably look incompetent.

THERAPIST: And if you make a relatively minor mistake?

CLIENT: If it's a minor mistake, no one will take much notice.

THERAPIST: OK. So now what you are saying is that there are different types of mistakes that could have different consequences?

CLIENT: Right.

THERAPIST: Look at your list of distortions (*pointing to Handout 5.2*). Do you recognize any distortion in your original thoughts?

CLIENT: Yes. Polarization. I'm seeing the situation in black-or-white terms.

THERAPIST: Right. It's not as simple as "Perfect performance equals competence, and a mistake equals incompetence." There are many possible outcomes, including a minor mistake's resulting in a successful outcome. . . . Now, let's look at the second automatic thought. It was "I really don't know what I'm doing." What supports this general conclusion that you don't know what you're doing?

CLIENT: Well, that general conclusion is not really true. I do know what I'm doing most of the time. Even in this area, I have a lot of knowledge. I may make a minor mistake, but I'm not likely to make any huge errors.

THERAPIST: If you look on the sheet of distortions, what might fit?

CLIENT: (*Pause*) . . . It looks like the second-to-last group. I'm minimizing my abilities to cope with the situation.

THERAPIST: Good. Let's go to the third thought: "I've got to make sure there are no mistakes." Do you recognize any distortion in this thought?

CLIENT: Unrealistic expectations?

THERAPIST: Why did you pick that one?

CLIENT: Well, I'm saying everything has to be perfect. There can't be any errors at all.

THERAPIST: Is that actually true?

CLIENT: Well, no. . . . Even though I'm not an expert in this area and may make a mistake, my mistakes are not likely to be serious. I am a competent lawyer, and I have a strong enough base of knowledge for handling this case in at least a satisfactory manner. This case probably is going to be a great opportunity for me to show others that I can handle this type of work.

Many types of questions can be used to expose blind spots and distortions. Handout 5.3 presents examples of different types of questions for the client's use.

Once core beliefs have been identified, they can be subjected to critical analyses or challenges. Systematically questioning beliefs with the guided discovery technique invariably exposes distortions in these beliefs. The following clinical vignette demonstrates how guided discovery is used to challenge one of Richard's core beliefs, identified earlier in this chapter.

THERAPIST: Let's look more closely at your belief that you have to perform perfectly to be loved, successful, and happy. Is this belief correct? Have you found any instances where this is not true?

CLIENT: Yes.

THERAPIST: When?

CLIENT: I love my wife, even though she doesn't do everything perfectly. And I love my kids, even though their behavior is far from perfect. No one can be perfect, and no one has to be perfect to be acceptable or loved. Truly loving someone is to love and accept them even with imperfections.

THERAPIST: And what about yourself? Do your wife and kids love and accept you, even though you don't do everything perfectly?

CLIENT: Yes. Thank God.

THERAPIST: And what about your boss? Do you have to perform perfectly to be accepted and successful at work?

CLIENT: No. I've made a number of mistakes—nothing major, of course. My work is actually more than acceptable to my boss. I am succeeding at work and getting raises, despite imperfect work performance.

THERAPIST: So what does all of this tell you about this belief?

CLIENT: The belief is not true, plain and simple.

Decatastrophizing

The decatastrophizing technique involves asking the client to focus on the worst-case scenario associated with a specific worry. Once a worst-case scenario is verbalized in full detail, the scenario can be examined for cognitive distortions.

As noted earlier, clients with GAD may overutilize worry as a way of cognitively avoiding emotional distress. Decatastrophizing can be used to confront such forms of cognitive avoidance. When an emotionally distressing cognition is avoided and not fully explored, it maintains its ability to evoke anxiety. The process of systematically exploring and questioning such cognitions invariably exposes distortions. When specific frightening thoughts, assumptions, beliefs, or images are openly stated, the client can be asked to make probability estimates for each. Often clients

CHALLENGING YOUR THOUGHTS

- Can I say that this statement is 100% true, without any exceptions?

- What is the likelihood or probability of this? (Rate twice: emotionally and objectively.)

- Does this statement fit with all of the available evidence?

- Am I ignoring any safety factors?

- Does this always apply? Are there conditions under which this might not apply?

- Is there a gray area (for polarization)?

- Is this based on fact or feeling? Have my feelings ever turned out to be wrong?

- How much control do I actually have in this situation? (Am I taking responsibility for things over which I have no control? Or am I ignoring aspects of the situation that I can control?)

- Is my expectation for this outcome realistic or even possible?

present thoughts such as "It would be the end of my marriage/career/life," "It would be intolerable," "I couldn't survive," or the like. In such instances, the client can be asked for ways he or she might cope with such extreme conditions. This can help the client realize the presence of coping abilities even with the worst-case scenarios. Occasionally, this part of the technique will expose skill deficiencies (e.g., assertiveness skills, time management, etc.) that will need to be corrected (see Chapter 8), so that feelings of mastery can be enhanced. The following clinical vignette demonstrates the decatastrophizing technique.

THERAPIST: It sounds like you were able to counteract the onset of some anxiety that you were experiencing in relation to a high-profile client on Tuesday.

CLIENT: Yeah. I made a mistake on a piece of advice that I gave him. I started to lose it when I realized the mistake, but I was able to use the challenges (*referring to Handout 5.3*) to calm myself down.

THERAPIST: Now that I see you have the gist of how to challenge these thoughts, I want to begin teaching you a technique called "decatastrophizing." This technique involves exploring your most catastrophic cognitions. Because this technique has you confronting your most frightening images, thoughts, assumptions, and beliefs, your anxiety level may climb very high at the start. As we continue to examine these cognitions, however, your level of anxiety will decrease. Would you like to use this example to learn this technique?

CLIENT: OK.

THERAPIST: You have down here that your first thoughts were "I made a mistake. This guy is going to think I'm a jerk." You recognized the errors in your thinking, and you were able to challenge those errors successfully. Good. For the purpose of learning this technique, however, let's do some "what if" imagining in relation to this situation. What if your worst-case scenario were to come true, and this guy actually did conclude that you are a jerk? Then what?

CLIENT: Oh, my God. That would be the worst. It would end my career.

THERAPIST: How much anxiety are you experiencing right now in relation to that thought?

CLIENT: I'm definitely anxious with that thought. I guess a 5. If that were true, my anxiety would probably go through the roof.

THERAPIST: What if this was a true fact . . . then what?

CLIENT: Disaster. I wouldn't recover. My career would be over.

THERAPIST: And what if your law career was over, then what?

CLIENT: My wife would leave me. My kids wouldn't have anything to do with me. I would end up all alone on the streets as one of these homeless people . . . totally depressed, unable to function, a leech on society.

THERAPIST: What do you think is the probability of all of this actually happening as the result of this guy thinking you are a jerk?

CLIENT: Well, this could happen.

THERAPIST: Yes, but what do you think is the *realistic* probability of this happening?

CLIENT: (*Pause*) . . . Close to zero, probably (*laughs slightly*).

THERAPIST: Why?

CLIENT: Well, this guy is important, but he's not that important. I do a lot of work for other clients who have been very pleased. I might lose the chance to work for this guy, and that would be disappointing, but he's not the end-all for my career.

THERAPIST: What about your wife leaving you? How likely is it that your wife would leave you if your law career ended?

CLIENT: That's not likely, either.

THERAPIST: Why not?

CLIENT: My wife loves me. She didn't marry me because I'm a lawyer. Actually, she tells me that she would be happy if I decided to change my career to something that was less labor-intensive.

THERAPIST: And what about your kids?

CLIENT: They'll continue to love me, because I love them and I'll do whatever is necessary to support them.

THERAPIST: And what about falling into a despondent state of depression?

CLIENT: That's your job to make sure that doesn't happen. I could always sue you for malpractice if you failed. I would be on easy street. . . . Just kidding!

THERAPIST: Are you trying to evoke my catastrophic cognitions? (*Both laugh.*)

It is important to remind the client that when catastrophic images, thoughts, assumptions, and beliefs are not followed through to their logical conclusions, their potential to evoke anxiety remains intact. The only way to weaken this potential is to confront these cognitions directly and evaluate them carefully. When probability estimates are realistic and distortions are countered, it is easier to let go of excessive worry. The consequent reduction in anxiety is a natural reinforcement for completing this process.

Step 3: Generating Alternative Viewpoints

Once the client can reliably recognize distorted cognitions and successfully challenge these distortions, the next step is to help him or her generate alternative viewpoints. Sometimes clients have no difficulty generating alternative perspectives. Other times they may be at a complete loss as to how to look at an event from another perspective. In the latter instance, the therapist's job is to help the client learn strategies for generating different viewpoints. Several strategies can be suggested: imagining the event from a third-person perspective; switching roles with another in the situation; viewing the event in a larger context or in a different time frame; asking about the presence of feelings other than anxiety; imagining best, worst, and then most realistic outcomes: and enlisting the help of others. We discuss each of these strategies next.

Imagining the Event from a Third-Person Perspective

The therapist can suggest that the client imagine the event from a third-person perspective. In other words, the client can imagine the event as seen by an emotionally uninvolved observer. Then the client can be encouraged to formulate different interpretations about the event from this more detached perspective. For example, a client fretted over a recent decline in the stock market. He worried that it signaled the beginning of another Great Depression, which would cause him to lose large sums of money. The client was encouraged to look at the decline as if he were an academic discussing the decline. From this analytic perspective, he recognized that the numerous gyrations in the market rarely foretold a major crash. Even when they represented a major downturn, they could be viewed as healthy cyclical corrections that also provided new investment opportunities.

Switching Roles

If the event involves an interaction with another person, the client can be asked to imagine switching roles, bearing in mind the other person's personality within this role. The client can also be asked to think of times when he or she has been in the other role. For example, another client was worried about how his boss viewed his performance. He assumed that his boss noticed each and every imperfection in his work. Here the client was told to imagine himself in his boss's role and to enact his boss's behavior in that role. With this exercise, the client recognized that his boss would have to work 24 hours a day, 7 days a week to examine each employee's work in such detail. Also, playing out the boss's attitude that the work needed to be adequate, instead of perfect, helped the client realize that his performance was probably viewed as more than adequate.

Changing the Frame

The therapist can suggest that the client look at an event from a larger context or within a different time frame. In other words, changing the frame surrounding an event may alter the significance of the event. For example, a client felt overwhelmed with worry over a number of specific problems at work. The therapist suggested viewing the events as if he was looking through a zoom lens. Zooming out from his tight focus on specific problems to a general overview helped the client clarify the relative importance of each specific problem. In another example, a client that feared his anxiety would spiral out of control (unending and without any natural containment) unless he avoided certain situations. The therapist suggested changing the time frame by fast-forwarding through the experience with the following questions: "How long do you think you would feel this way? And, how bad do you think the feelings would get? And then what?" This helped the client recognize that even the worst feelings are time-limited. If a client's knowledge about the natural ebb and flow of emotions is lacking, the therapist will need to provide corrective information (i.e., that anxiety naturally burns out and is replaced by a state of relaxation or fatigue after a certain point).

Taking Other Emotional Perspectives

A client sometimes ignores the presence of emotions other than fear or anxiety. The client can be helped to recognize the presence of other feelings with questions such as this: "Do you have any other feelings about this, like anger or relief?" When other emotions are identified, the therapist can ask the client to see the event from the perspective of the other emotion. For example, a client had knowledge that a member at his country club was spreading rumors about his financial situation. He worried that this would result in his being shunned and eventually excluded by other members. He was aware of anxious and fearful feelings. When queried for other feelings, the client became aware that he was also feeling angry with this particular member. He began to view this member's behavior as a problem to confront.

Imagining Extremes to Imagine the Middle

The therapist can suggest that the client imagine extreme outcomes (the worst and the best), and can then ask for the most realistic outcome within these extremes. When distortions are present, the client may find it easier to generate opposing viewpoints that are equally distorted before arriving at a realistic outcome.

Enlisting the Help of Others

The client can also enlist the help of trusted others to generate different perspectives. Instructing the client to present the concrete facts of an event, and then to ask others for their interpretation based on those facts, can elicit one or more alternative viewpoints. This can include seeking the therapist's viewpoint, of course.

Step 4: Creating Rational Responses and Hypothesis Testing

The last step in CR is to create rational responses that can be evaluated through real-life experience. The client is taught how to use the Rational Response Form to create a more adaptive interpretation of an event. The client is also taught how to set up a test for evaluating the validity of a newly developed interpretation.

Developing Rational Responses with the Rational Response Form

The Rational Response Form (see Handout 5.4) gives the client a structured way to integrate all of the information from the first three CR steps. The form provides areas for increasing awareness, challenging distorted cognitions, generating alternative viewpoints, and developing rational cognitive responses to trigger events. Filling out the form in session assists the client with learning

RATIONAL RESPONSE FORM

Trigger: _____

Cognitions (images, thoughts, assumptions, and/or beliefs): _____

_____

Strength of belief in cognitions (rate on a 0–8 scale): _____

Challenges: _____

_____

Types of thinking errors: _____

_____

Alternative viewpoints:
- Worst outcome: _____
- Best outcome: _____
- Most realistic outcome: _____

What effect does this thought or assumption have on the way I feel? _____

_____

Rational response:

Even though I feel that _____ is true,
(thought or assumption)

the reality is that _____.
(answers to challenges and alternative viewpoints)

how to use the forms on his or her own. The following clinical vignette (again, the client is Richard) provides an example of how to help the client through this process.

THERAPIST: I see on your log that you had an episode of worry that was spurred by a pimple that you noticed on your skin. You wrote down that your thought was "Cancer." Is that thought still getting triggered by the pimple?

CLIENT: Yes.

THERAPIST: Why don't we use this situation as an example of how to use the Rational Response Form (*gives Handout 5.4 to client*)?

CLIENT: OK.

THERAPIST: Write down "Pimple" on the top line next to "Trigger," and "Cancer" on the second line next to "Cognitions." How strongly do you believe that this thought is true?

CLIENT: Well, I'm probably being ridiculous. There's probably very little chance that this is cancer.

THERAPIST: Is that what you think on a rational level?

CLIENT: Yes. I know this thought probably isn't rational, but it still scares me. I don't really see how this form is going to help.

THERAPIST: It sounds like you're feeling a bit frustrated.

CLIENT: Yes.

THERAPIST: Is that because even though you may know something does not make sense on a rational level, you are still feeling as if it did make sense?

CLIENT: Yes, that's it.

THERAPIST: Tuning in to your gut or emotional reaction, how would you rate the strength of this thought "Cancer"?

CLIENT: I would say a 7.

THERAPIST: Write down that rating on the next line. . . . As you can see, you are rating the validity of this thought very differently, depending upon whether you are using your rational side or your emotional side. One problem right now is that these two sides are separate. They stand independent of one another. The purpose of this form is to help you to integrate these two sides and arrive at one viewpoint.

CLIENT: OK.

THERAPIST: All right, let's start to challenge this thought. What is the objective evidence that supports this thought?

CLIENT: Well, it hurts. It looks funny.

THERAPIST: Anything else?

CLIENT: Not really. Well, I read an article about the incidence of skin cancer increasing.

THERAPIST: Is that a piece of objective evidence that supports the notion that this pimple is cancer?

CLIENT: Well, no. Actually, what they described as signs and symptoms of skin cancer doesn't really fit with what this pimple looks like. I guess I don't have any other evidence.

THERAPIST: It sounds like the information that you read provided evidence to contradict the idea that this pimple is cancerous. Is that right?

CLIENT: Yeah, I guess it did.

THERAPIST: Do you have any other evidence that this is not cancer?

CLIENT: Let me think. . . . I had a pimple like this about 6 months ago. It went away eventually. Come to think of it, I had this same thought then. . . . But what if I was just lucky that time, and now the real thing is occurring?

THERAPIST: Does that fit with what you read in that article?

CLIENT: No.

THERAPIST: Why not?

CLIENT: The pimple looks the same. If it wasn't cancer then, it's not likely to be cancer now.

THERAPIST: What do you think is the objective probability that this is cancer?

CLIENT: Nearly 0%.

THERAPIST: OK. Write down under "Challenges" the objective probability of this being cancer and your list of reasons for this rating. . . . .What kinds of distortions can you recognize?

CLIENT: It looks like I'm catastrophizing and making faulty estimates.

THERAPIST: OK. Write that down in the section labeled "Types of thinking errors." Can you think of an alternative viewpoint?

CLIENT: I'm fine. I have an annoying pimple again. It'll go away eventually.

THERAPIST: Write that down. . . . Now I want you to consider what the worst possible outcome could be, given the objective evidence.

CLIENT: Let's see. . . . Given the objective evidence, the pimple could get infected, and I'll go to the doctor and have it lanced. Maybe I'll be put on antibiotics.

THERAPIST: And the best possible outcome?

CLIENT: It goes away after several days.

THERAPIST: What's most realistic?

CLIENT: It goes away after several days.

THERAPIST: Write all of that down. . . . How could you summarize all of this in the last statement at the end of the page?

CLIENT: Even though I'm worried that this pimple means I have cancer, the reality that the symptoms associated with this pimple are not those that occur with cancer. I've had a pimple like this in the past. This pimple will go away, just like the other went away.

THERAPIST: OK. Now rate the strength of your belief, using your emotional side, that this thought is true.

CLIENT: It's about a 3.

THERAPIST: And how are you feeling?

CLIENT: Better. Less anxious.

THERAPIST: Good. If you are feeling a decrease, the form is doing its job in helping you to weaken the emotional impact of these thoughts.

The client can be instructed to begin using this form any time images, thoughts, assumptions, or beliefs associated with worry episodes are identified. It is best if the client can work through the Rational Response Form when the worry episode occurs.

Clients sometimes expect that if they work through this form once or twice, they will feel better any time they are confronted with the trigger situation. It is important to remind such clients that these cognitive patterns are deeply ingrained, habitual ways of interpreting reality. As such, they can be viewed as bad habits. Being able to break a bad habit successfully on one or two occasions does not mean that the habit is broken permanently. To do the latter, one must purposely and repeatedly break the habit on numerous occasions. (If the client ever has had to unlearn a bad habit in playing a sport or a musical instrument, or has ever tried to stop smoking, the client will have concrete experience with the slow, deliberate, and arduous effort required to eliminate any bad habit.) The client can be reminded that the amount of effort expended on these exercises is related to the amount and rate of progress.

Hypothesis Testing

When newly developed rational responses leave the client less than convinced, experiments can be set up to test these new interpretations. Hypothesis testing involves setting up specific conditions in real life where different interpretations can be evaluated. After the experiment is conducted, the therapist and client examine the concrete data to determine whether the different interpretations are either supported or refuted. Real-life experiments that test various hypotheses often prove to be the most powerful agents for solidifying change in cognition.

Using the incident of Richard's daughter at the playground presented earlier in this chapter, the therapist and Richard identify two hypotheses. The first is Richard's view of the situation: that the playground is a dangerous place for his daughter. The second interpretation is that the playground is a fairly safe place for her to play. The real-life test is to have Richard take his daughter to the playground three times each week over the next 2 weeks; to allow her to play uninterrupted until she is tired (up to 2 hours); and to observe and record the outcomes for his daughter and all of the other children at the playground. After observing and discussing with the therapist that the kids are simply having fun and are not getting hurt (except for an occasional scuffed knee), Richard is able to begin relaxing in this situation.

POSITIVE IMAGERY

The positive imagery technique is based on Lang's (1985) notion that somatic activation of emotion occurs by way of imagery. By strengthening abilities to harness and develop control over internal images, the client can voluntarily produce different types of central nervous system activation through vivid imagery. Once fully trained, the client can use imagery that activates parasympathetic activity to counteract images that activate sympathetic activity. The positive imagery technique could also be conceptualized as a relaxation skill technique. It has been included in the cognitive component chapter of this book, however, because this technique uses mental images to manipulate physiological activity rather than directly. Positive imagery has been used as an alternative relaxation skill in applied relaxation (AR). It has also been used to imagine positive coping responses to develop an alternative historical record within the self-control desensitization (S-CD) technique. (Both AR and S-CD are described in Chapter 6.)

To develop clients' imaging capabilities, clients are instructed to imagine neutral or relaxing scenes twice a day throughout the training period. The scenes in Table 5.3 are examples of what may be used. The therapist should instruct the client to focus on each of the senses (sight, sound, smell, touch, and/or taste) and his or her internal bodily sensations while imagining each scene. Therapists and clients can modify these scenes or use other scenes for training. Therapists can ask clients to describe scenes in which they feel extremely relaxed. These descriptions should also incorporate applicable experiences of the five senses and internal bodily sensations.

An environment where the client will not be distracted is best for practicing. Specific beginning and ending times (e.g., 5 minutes) should be set for each image. The client should attempt to initiate and maintain vivid images throughout the duration of each 5-minute exercise. In addition, the client should attempt to terminate the image completely at the end of each exercise.

Following each imagery practice, clients should rate the vividness of their mental imagery, as well as the degree of relaxation during imagery, on the Positive Imagery Rating Form (see Handout 5.5). The goal is for clients to consistently achieve ratings of 6–8 for applicable items on the vividness scale and ratings of 6–8 on the relaxation scale. Training is then complete for the use of imagery in AR or S-CD.

WORRY EXPOSURE

Borkovec and Inz (1990) made the suggestion, based on their research, that worry is an active attempt to avoid and control emotional distress evoked by particular images. Avoiding images by worrying, however, is an ineffective strategy for long-term anxiety reduction, because worrying only temporarily reduces distress. An association of a direct personal threat with a particular image remains intact and ready to evoke more episodes of worry, as long as the affect associated with that image is avoided. A "phobic" type of response to such images can develop with excessive avoidance. For these reasons, worry exposure may be a particularly important component of treatment. Worry exposure teaches clients to accept, tolerate, and eventually habituate to emotional reactions associated with certain images. A long-term reduction in anxiety associated with these images is achieved by directly facing the images and habituating to the emotional responses associated with them.

Worry exposure consists of teaching the client to accept, rather than avoid, resist, or fight, the emotional distress associated with certain images. The client purposely exposes him- or herself for extended periods of time to various images, without avoiding or escaping the full emotional impact of those images. Such avoidance can be overt (behavioral avoidance) or covert (e.g., worry,

TABLE 5.3. Positive Imagery Scripts

Scene 1: Drinking cold lemonade on a hot summer day

You are at a country fair on a sunny, hot summer day. Your legs are tired, and your feet ache slightly from all the walking. The ground is dry and dusty and feels hard under your feet. There is a slight breeze as you walk. It makes the droplets of sweat on your neck and brow and around your lips feel cool, but your mouth and throat feel parched. You smell the aroma of hot dogs, hamburgers, and fries as you walk toward a stand selling refreshments. As you reach the stand, you hear the food searing on the grill and frying in the heavy grease. As you wait to order your drink, other people line up behind you. You feel the air go still as they block out even the slightest breeze. You order a lemonade and then watch the young boy prepare it. He puts the tall white paper cup before you. You raise your hand to grasp the drink and feel the coolness of the paper cup in your hand. As you look into the cup, you see the pale lemon-yellow color of the drink broken up by pieces of clear ice. As you plunk down your change on the Formica counter with one hand, the other hand raises the cup to your lips. You tilt your head back and spill the cool, wet drink into your mouth. All of your senses are focused on the sweet, tart lemon flavor slightly puckering your mouth. You feel the cold ice cubes against your lips as the cool liquid enters your mouth and cascades down to the back of your throat. You feel your body cooling as you swallow repeatedly. You pull your head straight and lower your hand with the cup in it for a brief break. You see others relishing their drinks and food. You return your attention to your lemonade and resume until you drink your fill.

Scene 2: Walking through the woods on a fall day

You are walking on a path in the woods on a clear, cool morning in the fall. Your eyes feast on the intense colors around you. The oranges, reds, yellows, browns, and greens of the foliage wake up your senses. The sky is a deep blue. The contrast of the sky with the kaleidoscope of leaves makes the leaves' colors even more vivid. The air feels crisp, cool, and dry against your cheeks and lips. Your fingers are beginning to ache from the cold. You shove your hands into your coat pockets. The softness of the lining inside comforts your hands. As you walk along, you hear the rustling of the leaves underfoot. Your feet feel cushioned by the fresh layer of newly fallen leaves. You spot a pretty, bright red leaf with flashes of yellow on the ground. You stop walking to bend down and pick it up. You notice the smell of the earth. As you stand back up, you feel the leaf's thin, firm stem and the damp, rubbery texture of its body. You run your fingers along the veins. You resume walking and decide to pick up your pace. You begin to feel your heart beating and your respiration quicken with each step. Your cheeks and hands start to flush and feel warm. You feel invigorated and experience a sense of pleasure in being alive. You continue to walk briskly for a brief period. Eventually, your pace returns to normal. You feel your heart and breath slowly readjusting to this more relaxed pace.

Scene 3: Taking a hot bath

You hear water surging into the tub as you take off your clothes. You feel cold air against your body. Your muscles tense, and a shiver rushes through your body. Tiny bumps rise on your skin. You quickly step on the soft, thick, plush green rug to take the chill off your feet. You touch the wall to steady yourself while you turn off the water. The wall tiles feel hard and cold against your fingers. Putting your foot into the water, you feel its warmth surrounding your toes, arch, and ankle. You quickly put your other foot in and sit down. Warm, moist steam rises from the water into your face. A thin film of moisture forms on your brow and upper lip. You slowly recline into the water, letting it wash over your entire body. You hear the water gently lapping against the sides of the tub. A bar of soap nearby emanates a subtle, sweet smell. The water feels warm and soothing. It loosens your muscles. You feel your muscles unwinding and relaxing . . . letting go of all tension. You feel comfortable and deeply relaxed. Pleasant images wander through your mind.

POSITIVE IMAGERY RATING FORM

Brief description of image: _____

	Image vividness ratings								
	None			Moderate				Extreme	
Visual	0	1	2	3	4	5	6	7	8
Auditory	0	1	2	3	4	5	6	7	8
Tactile	0	1	2	3	4	5	6	7	8
Taste	0	1	2	3	4	5	6	7	8
Olfactory	0	1	2	3	4	5	6	7	8
Visceral	0	1	2	3	4	5	6	7	8

Relaxation scale

−8	−7	−6	−5	−4	−3	−2	−1	0	1	2	3	4	5	6	7	8
Extreme increase in tension								No change								Extreme increase in relaxation

distraction, punishment, problem solving). Accepting and tolerating emotional responses allow the habituation process to occur. Through this process, the association of fear and avoidance responses with particular images can be extinguished. The ultimate goal of worry exposure is for the individual to experience the images simply as images and not as realistic representations of actual threats to his or her well-being.

There are six steps in the implementation of this procedure:

1. Emotionally distressing images evocative of worry must be identified. This can be done through self-monitoring or through the vertical descent method mentioned earlier in this chapter.
2. The images are ranked according to their anxiety-provoking level (0–8) on a hierarchy. This hierarchy is used to select items for graded exposure exercises.
3. The client is instructed to use subjective units of distress (SUDs) ratings during the exposures. Levels of distress are rated on a 0–100 scale, with 0 representing no distress, 25 mild distress, 50 moderate distress, 75 severe distress, and 100 extreme distress (see Handout 5.6, Worry Exposure SUDs Rating Form).
4. To begin, the item with the lowest-level rating from the anxiety hierarchy is selected for an exposure.
5. The purpose of the initial exposure is to collect a detailed narrative of the image from the client. At the beginning of the exposure, the therapist sets the scene and then asks the client to describe in as much detail as possible what is happening in the image. The client is instructed to use all of his or her senses to make the image as vivid as possible. The description should include physiological sensations experienced by the client while imaging. The therapist is to stay alert for any signs of cognitive or behavioral avoidance of the image throughout the client's narration. If any avoidance is noticed, the therapist should gently remind the client to refocus on the image. This narrative is either tape-recorded or written out by either the therapist or the client.
6. Subsequent exposures are conducted by having the client read or listen to this narration in full. With each exposure to the narration, the client is reminded to maintain his or her focus on the frightening images without allowing any cognitive or behavioral avoidance. The exposures are conducted in tight succession, with SUDs ratings collected every 30 seconds throughout. The imagining procedure continues until the client's SUDs levels reach half the level noted at the beginning of the procedure.

Step 6 is repeated until the anxiety level for that hierarchy item drops to 0 or 1. The next item on the hierarchy is then selected, and Steps 5 and 6 are repeated until all items on the hierarchy drop to 0 or 1.

The following clinical vignette demonstrates this procedure with Richard.

THERAPIST: Today we are going to concentrate on a technique called "worry exposure." This technique allows you to become desensitized to images that distress you. When people are repeatedly exposed to upsetting images for long enough, they will no longer be upset by the images.

HANDOUT 5.6. Worry Exposure SUDS Ratings Form

WORRY EXPOSURE SUDS RATINGS FORM

Day/date/time: _____

Image: _____

Beginning level (0–100): ____

    30 seconds: ____   30 seconds: ____

    30 seconds: ____   30 seconds: ____

    30 seconds: ____   30 seconds: ____

    30 seconds: ____   30 seconds: ____

    30 seconds: ____   30 seconds: ____

    30 seconds: ____   30 seconds: ____

    30 seconds: ____   30 seconds: ____

    30 seconds: ____   30 seconds: ____

    30 seconds: ____   30 seconds: ____

    30 seconds: ____   30 seconds: ____

    30 seconds: ____   30 seconds: ____

    30 seconds: ____   30 seconds: ____

    30 seconds: ____   30 seconds: ____

    30 seconds: ____   Ending Level: ____

Note. Based on Craske, Barlow, and O'Leary (1992).

The process is similar to what everyone experiences when we see disasters played and replayed in the news. Initially, images of the disaster are very upsetting and disturbing. We are both attracted to finding out more about the disaster and repelled by the emotional distress associated with the horrific images. We all have questions and concerns about the possibility of personally experiencing such an event. Over time, emotional reactivity to images of the disaster fades. This occurs with continued exposures to the horrific events, in conjunction with the concrete experiences of everyday. Eventually, the disaster images are viewed as sad and unfortunate, but they are no longer upsetting. Have you ever noticed this process occurring within yourself?

CLIENT: Yes. I noticed this with the Oklahoma City bombings and 9/11.

THERAPIST: With all the media coverage, many people have gone through this process with these events. Worry exposure is a technique where you face the disturbing images that evoke your worry.

Most people experience an increase in their anxiety as they begin to focus on frightening images. You also are likely to experience this increase. Individuals with anxiety disorders sometimes fear that once anxiety is activated, it continues to progress to more intense levels endlessly. But the fact is that emotional reactions like anxiety eventually dissipate. You may want to stop the anxiety-provoking images to prevent emotions from spiraling out of control. But if you do, you'll never experience the natural endpoint to distress associated with anxiety-provoking images.

Forced exposure to these images will allow you to build up tolerance to feelings of anxiety. But with this technique, you must allow yourself to experience the full impact of the emotional distress associated with disturbing images, until it naturally fades each time. Then, as you repeat the exposure to these images, you will notice that your strongest emotional reactions grow less and less intense as you "habituate" or get used to the images. This will be uncomfortable, but I will be here with you. You also will experience concrete events around you as unchanged, stable, and safe. The physiological mobilization or arousal associated with these images will eventually also fade, because it will be experientially recognized as unnecessary. After repeated presentations of the images, you will notice that you experience the images simply as negative images with little personal significance.

In the last session, we identified many images that trigger worry for you. Today we will use the lowest-level item from the anxiety hierarchy to practice this technique. How does that sound?

CLIENT: OK.

THERAPIST: You had an image of your boss looking at your memo with dissatisfaction and imagined him thinking, "I've got to get rid of this guy." You rated your anxiety with this item at 3. Does that seem accurate to you right now?

CLIENT: Yes.

THERAPIST: OK. We will begin by creating a detailed and fully developed narrative of this image. Often other images spontaneously occur during this process. It is important to fully explore and describe each of these images during the development of the narrative. During repeated exposure exercises, you will be listening to a taped playback of this narrative. Before we begin working on the narrative, however, I want to prepare you for what you may experience while we work on this narrative and during the exposures. When emotional reactions are tolerated, the individual recognizes that the negative outcomes represented in images never, or very rarely, occur. You will notice that your anxiety associated with particular images naturally climaxes and then dissipates. It is important to continue with whatever images occur during these exercises, and to repeat these images until you experience this dissipation in your level of anxiety. Are you ready to begin?

CLIENT: Sure.

THERAPIST: OK. I am going to have you close your eyes and imagine this situation. You noted that you were at work and had noticed an error in a memo sent to your boss right before this image occurred. I'm going to start by having you imagine yourself in this situation and experiencing this image again. While you are imagining this situation, I want you to talk out loud, describing everything in the image. I want you to describe every detail—everything you are seeing, hearing, touching, tasting, and/or smelling. Describe everything that you and others are doing and saying. I also want you to describe everything that you are feeling while you are experiencing this image. Describe all of your bodily sensations. I will be tape-recording this portion of the session. OK?

CLIENT: OK.

THERAPIST: (*Starts recording*) Now, close your eyes. . . . Picture yourself in your office at work . . . Imagine yourself sitting in your chair at your desk. . . . Picture the lighting, the walls, the desk, your chair, the work papers around you, your phone, and other things on top of your desk. . . . Feel the chair that you sit in and the desk in front of you as you lean forward to review your memo. . . . Feel the crisp paper in your hands. . . . As you begin to read the memo, you notice a minor error in the memo that you just sent off to your boss. . . . Just continue with the image and tell me what's happening.

CLIENT: I see my boss looking at my memo. He's dissatisfied and disgusted. He thinks, "I've got to get rid of this guy." I feel tension in my back and neck. My chest is tight. I picture him with the other partners at review time. They disparage my work and mutually agree to toss me out of the firm. I feel panicky. I see myself interviewing at other firms along with huge numbers of candidates. I'm feeling overwhelmed and distressed. Our financial situation deteriorates. There's not enough money to cover expenses. I go to work at a fast-food restaurant, trying to make ends meet. My wife goes back to work. She's exhausted and irritable. My kids are unhappy. There's no money for toys. We barely scrape by. We sell our house and move into a small apartment. It looks a mess. We don't have time or energy to keep it up. We are exhausted, and our kids are neglected. My wife and kids look ragged. No one visits us. We're shunned by what used to be our friends. We are isolated and desperate. There's no way out.

THERAPIST: (*Turns off the tape recorder*) OK. Now I'm going to replay the tape. I want you to close your eyes again and reinvolve yourself in the images as much as possible. At different points throughout the tape, I will be asking you to rate you level of distress on a 0–100 scale, with 0 representing no distress, 25 mild distress, 50 moderate distress, 75 severe distress, and 100 extreme distress. These ratings are called "SUDs," which stands for "subjective units of distress." I will ask you to make SUDs ratings throughout the exercise. Rate your anxiety quickly, and then return to the images. These ratings will allow both of us to observe how your level of anxiety changes over time. Are you ready to listen to the tape?

CLIENT: OK.

THERAPIST: Before we start, give me a SUDs rating right now.

CLIENT: 50.

THERAPIST: All right. Here we go again. (*Therapist writes down the rating and starts playing the tape, asking for SUDs ratings approximately every 30 seconds.*)

The therapist should replay the tape or reread the written narrative (if there is no recording) until the therapist sees significant decrements in the SUDs ratings over the course of several exposures. As a rule of thumb, the client's highest SUDs levels at the beginning should be cut in half by the end of the procedure. Only then should the therapist stop repeating the narrative. After this point, the therapist may want to conduct CR exercises related to the image(s) as well.

The tape or written narrative should be given to the client for between-session assignments of worry exposure. The client should be instructed to make SUDs ratings before, during, and after these exercises on Handout 5.6. It is important to instruct the client to abstain from any type of avoidance of the images (e.g., worry, distraction, problem solving) during the exposures. CR exercises with the images should occur only after SUDs levels are consistently 50% lower than the initial levels.

IMPROVING PROBLEM ORIENTATION

Ladouceur, Blais, Freeston, and Dugas (1998) found that problem-solving skills are unrelated to excessive worry associated with GAD. Rather, worry is associated with positive problem-solving behaviors such as problem-focused coping behaviors and information-seeking strategies (Davey, Hampton, Farrell, & Davidson, 1992). Deficiencies appear in the confidence levels associated with problem solving and in the sense of personal control over the problem-solving process (Davey, 1994a, 1994b). Based on this and their own research, Dugas, Gagnon, Ladouceur, and Freeston (1998) suggest that the difficulties may lie in the individual's orientation to the problem and tolerance of uncertainty.

Dugas et al. (1998) suggest that these difficulties can be corrected with the following procedures. First, the client's worry problems are categorized as pertaining to either immediate or improbable events. Worry exposure is suggested for excessive worry associated with improbable events. For excessive worry associated with immediate events, they suggest the following procedures: training clients to stay focused on key elements of the immediate problem, and to ignore minor details associated with that problem; restructuring cognitions associated with beliefs regarding the benefits of worry and needs for certainty; increasing clients' abilities to cope with uncertain outcomes. Although Dugas et al. (1998) do not make specific recommendations on how to increase clients' abilities to cope, this might be accomplished with AR or diaphragmatic breathing (see Chapter 6) or through *in vivo* exposure (see Chapter 7). Since these treatment recommendations have not yet been empirically tested for their effectiveness, they are presented in this section as potentially beneficial in the treatment of GAD.

COST–BENEFIT ANALYSIS OF COPING RESPONSES

To increase awareness of distortions in the perceived costs and benefits of certain coping responses, the therapist can conduct an analysis of these responses in relation to specific stimulus events. To conduct the analysis, the therapist should instruct the client to draw four quadrants like those in Handout 5.7. The four quadrants are headed as follows: "Advantages of [coping response] when [stimulus] occurs," "Disadvantages of [coping response] when [stimulus] occurs," "Advantages of [alternative response] when [stimulus] occurs," and "Disadvantages of [alternative response] when [stimulus] occurs." Both short- and long-term advantages and disadvantages should be fully explored from a rational perspective (guided discovery or the Rational Response Form may need to be used with some items). This analysis increases awareness of the costs of excessive and unnecessary coping responses, and the benefits of letting go of these responses. This analysis is helpful in identifying both cognitive and behavioral coping responses that are excessive and/or unnecessary.

SCHEDULED WORRY TIME

By the time clients reach treatment, worry has often become associated with a multitude of stimuli. The goal of "scheduled worry time" is to weaken automatic associations between the three components of the worry process and external and internal stimuli. Scheduled worry time inhibits the generalization of worry to new stimuli and promotes extinction of existing associations of worry with stimuli. Borkovec, Wilkinson, Folensbee, and Lerman (1983) originally conceptualized scheduled worry time as a stimulus control technique for containing worry and obtained positive results. More recently, this technique has been categorized as a response prevention technique, with worry conceptualized as a cognitive response that can be prevented. This method places tight restrictions on where and when worry is permitted, and so enables clients to regain control over the worry process and the stimuli that evoke worry.

Many clients with GAD believe that their worry is necessary (e.g., problem solving to avoid a future threat). Thus, for them, just giving up the worry is very difficult. With scheduled worry time, the goal is not to give up the worry, but to delay it until a later point in time. As a result, it may be easier for the client to do this rather than try to give up or challenge worry altogether.

COST–BENEFIT ANALYSIS OF COPING RESPONSES

Advantages of _____ (coping response)	Disadvantages of _____ (coping response)
Advantages of _____ (alternative response)	Disadvantages of _____ (alternative response)

Scheduled worry time involves asking clients to set specified times and locations for worry. If clients find themselves worrying at other times, they are instructed to disengage from the worry and save the worry for a scheduled worry time.

There are four steps (see Table 5.4) in the implementation of this procedure. The first step is to use the treatment version of the Worry Episode Log for identifying worrisome thoughts to be delayed. The second step is to establish a daily 30- to 60-minute worry period at a specified time and location (e.g., on the train ride home after work). The third step is practicing delay and postponement of worry until the scheduled worry time. This is done by "letting go" of worry through refocusing attention on aspects of the external environment (e.g., sensations, sights, sounds, tasks at hand, a conversation, etc.).

In presenting this step of the technique, it is extremely important that the client understand what "letting go" of worry involves. The client's attitude toward worry needs to be one of accepting and relocating worry, rather than fighting to actively suppress or get rid of worry. Worry concerns future and/or past events and not the present. The client's intentional refocusing of attention on stimuli in the immediate external environment maximizes the chances that the client will be able to "let go" of worry, as opposed to fully engaging with it. The client is to notice and accept worry and then delay or postpone attention to the worry until a different time and place. This point is extremely important, because research indicates that active attempts to control or intentionally suppress worry increase its frequency (Wegner, Schneider, Carter, & White, 1987; Clark, Ball, & Pape, 1991). Throughout the exercises, worry is accepted simply as worry. Any purposeful efforts to suppress worry are suspended. Again, the attitude is one of accepting, delaying, and relocating worry, rather than fighting worry.

The fourth step is for the client to use the 30- to 60-minute scheduled worry time exclusively for worry. During this period of time, the client brings all of the stored worries into awareness. The client is encouraged to use scheduled worry times to intentionally expose him- or herself to images that evoke worry (see "Worry Exposure"), and/or to subject the worry to critical analyses through CR exercises on thoughts, assumptions, and/or beliefs (see "Creating Rational Responses and Hypothesis Testing") and cost–benefit exercises (see "Cost–Benefit Analysis of Coping Responses").

TABLE 5.4. Implementing Scheduled Worry Time

1. Client identifies specific worries with the Worry Episode Log (for Treatment)
2. With client, set a specific time and place for a daily 30- to 60-minute worry period.
3. Teach, and have client practice, how to "let go" of worry by refocusing attention on the immediate external environment.
4. Client uses scheduled time for worry.

Note. Based on Borkovec, Wilkinson, Folensbee, and Lerman (1983).

WORRY-FREE ZONES

Boutselis (see Borkovec, Alcaine, & Behar, 2004) developed the technique of "worry-free zones." This technique is similar to the scheduled worry time technique. In both techniques, worry is delayed or postponed under certain conditions, and the same approach for the delay and postponement of worry is utilized. With the worry-free zone technique, however, a specific time in a specific location is designated as a worry-free period. Over time, this worry-free zone is expanded to include longer periods of time and an increasing number of locations.

PROBLEMATIC CLIENT RESPONSES TO COGNITIVE TECHNIQUES

A client may resist questioning his or her perceptions, or may appear to be highly invested in maintaining certain perceptions. In this instance, the therapist may find that questioning the client's perception results in the client's becoming more and more vehemently in favor of maintaining his or her worries. Rather than persisting with the Socratic method of questioning the client's interpretation, the therapist can stop to look for the grain of truth in the client's interpretation and join with the client on this point. Once a client feels that the therapist understands and acknowledges the "emotional" validity of the perception, the client often then is more willing to begin exploring the "objective" validity of the perception.

Once a client understands how to use the rational response form, he or she may prematurely suspend filling out these forms consistently and systematically. It is very important that the therapist keep clients on task with these assignments. These techniques must be over-learned to be truly useful in high-anxiety situations. Only when clients report that they notice themselves mentally going through the challenges automatically under high-anxiety conditions can the practice of manually filling out the forms be suspended. The goal is for the challenges to become automatic responses.

A client may worry during exposures rather than exposing him- or herself to the images that generate worry. On occasion, a client misunderstands the purpose of the worry exposure and engages in pure worry during these exercises. It is very important that the therapist be crystal clear that the client is not to engage in prolonged periods of worry during these. Prolonged bouts of worry will intensify rather than diminish worry. The therapist must make it extremely clear that the exposures are to the frightening images that evoke worry. The therapist should instruct the client to focus on the images and not avoid the images by worrying. If worry is noticed during an exposure, the client should try (as best as he or she is able) to suspend and/or delay the worry and refocus attention on the upsetting images. It is the prolonged exposures to the images, rather than to worry, that weakens the link between the images and the worry process.

CHAPTER SIX

Treating the Physiological Component

The increased physical arousal associated with GAD involves multiple physiological systems, including the nervous, cardiovascular, respiratory, and gastrointestinal systems. Hypervigilance accompanies this state of high arousal. Physical arousal, however, can be voluntarily altered with training in relaxation skills. In essence, this training enables clients to shift physical functions voluntarily toward those that naturally occur in a relaxed state. In the first part of this chapter, we present three methods for purposefully achieving a relaxed state; two different protocols for training progressive muscular relaxation (PMR) and one protocol for training diaphragmatic breathing (DB) are provided. In the second part of this chapter, we discuss two techniques that utilize relaxation skills to interrupt the spiraling process of worry: self-control desensitization (S-CD) and applied relaxation (AR). Table 6.1 lists the specific techniques covered in this chapter. In the last section of this chapter, we discuss problems that may be encountered with relaxation exercises and/or the techniques that utilize them. Potential solutions to these problems are offered.

TABLE 6.1. Techniques That Target the Physiological Component of GAD

Progressive Muscular Relaxation (PMR)	Diaphragmatic breathing (DB)
15-muscle-group PMR	Self-control desensitization (S-CD)
Alternative version of PMR	Applied relaxation (AR)

PROGRESSIVE MUSCULAR RELAXATION (PMR)

Edmund Jacobson originally developed PMR in 1929. Many versions of this exercise have been created since then and have been used in numerous treatment outcome studies for GAD (e.g., Barlow et al., 1984; Barlow, Rapee, & Brown, 1992; Borkovec & Costello, 1993; Öst & Breitholtz, 2000). Two versions of PMR—a 15-muscle-group PMR exercise and an alternative version of PMR typically used in AR (discussed later in this chapter)—are included in this section. PMR directly targets muscular tension associated with episodes of general anxiety. Heart and respiration rates, as well as muscular tension, can be reduced with these exercises. The exercises not only increase awareness of the buildup of muscle tension at earlier and earlier stages, but give the client a way to counteract these tensions.

The 15-Muscle-Group PMR Exercise

This first version of the PMR exercise has two steps. The first step has two parts: The therapist (1) teaches the client how to tense and relax 15 different muscle groups and then (2) trains the client to systematically tense and relax those muscle groups within the context of a scripted relaxation exercise. The second step repeats the training, but with one major modification to the relaxation exercise—the 15 muscle groups are relaxed only. Through this training, the client learns to intentionally achieve a deep state of relaxation throughout his or her body. The exercise, as described below, is based on the version by Klosko & Sanderson (1999).

PMR is a skill that can be learned through regular practice. A quiet, dimly lit room is an ideal environment for practicing the exercise. The therapist's office can be arranged to provide this type of setting. Initially, the exercise should be practiced in a semireclined position, with eyes closed and all parts of the body fully supported when relaxed. Later, the exercises should be practiced under increasingly typical daytime conditions (e.g., sitting up, lights on, TV or radio on). To master PMR, two daily practices are ideal. One daily practice may be sufficient; however, less practice is likely to result in problems with mastering this skill.

An audiotape of the exercise should be given to the client at the first training session. Taping the initial in-session exercise is an easy way to create the tape. The purpose of the tape is to familiarize the client with the exercise. It is to be used within the first 2 weeks, only; the client should attempt the exercise without the tape thereafter.

Step 1: The Tension-Release PMR Exercise

Part 1: Training Muscle Tensing and Relaxing. Training begins with a description of the differences between muscular tension and relaxation. This includes a demonstration of how to "let go" and how to create muscular tension with a specific muscle group. The therapist then demonstrates how to tense and release tension in 15 different muscle groups.

The therapist explains that when a muscle is deeply relaxed, it feels extremely loose and limp (similar to cooked spaghetti). All tension and resistance within the muscle are released. The therapist uses his or her own body to demonstrate complete relaxation of the muscles in one arm by lifting this arm with his or her hand and then letting it go so that it drops like dead weight. The therapist then asks the client to do the same, making sure that the client understands how to relax or to let go of muscle tension completely. To encourage the release of tension, the therapist can instruct the client to take a deep breath and then, as he or she exhales, to relax the muscle group slowly. As the client relaxes that muscle group, the client can think of the word "relax."

The therapist then explains and demonstrates how to tense 15 specific muscle groups (see Table 6.2). When showing the client how to tense the different muscle groups, the therapist can ask whether the tensions are similar to those that are experienced during episodes of worry. If the client reports a different type of tension within a muscle group, the instructions can be modified to accommodate those tensions. It is not necessary that the client follow these instructions exactly. The exercise can be done in a number of different ways. The important point is that the client feels tension in each muscle group. If any pain is experienced while tensing a particular muscle group, the client should be instructed to focus on existing tension in that muscle group and to refrain from adding tension. When clients initially attempt to tense a muscle group, they often tense more than that one muscle group. If this occurs, it is important to call attention to this fact and have the client practice tensing only that one group, while leaving the other muscle groups in a relatively relaxed state.

The client is then encouraged to tense and relax each muscle group along with the therapist. The creation of tension in each group is immediately followed by the full release of tension in that same group. To produce tension in the scalp and upper forehead, the eyebrows are elevated to create wrinkles in the forehead. While the client is releasing the tensions, the therapist can give

TABLE 6.2. Tensing Instructions for 15-Muscle-Group Progressive Muscular Relaxation (PMR)

Muscle group	Tensing instructions
Scalp/upper forehead	"Raise your eyebrows to wrinkle your forehead."
Lower forehead	"Push your eyebrows down into a frown."
Eyes	"Close your eyes tightly (but not too tightly with contacts)."
Mouth	"Purse your lips."
Jaw	"Push your chin out and pull the corners of your mouth back."
Back of neck	"Lower your chin until it almost touches your collar bone."
Shoulders	"Raise your shoulders up close to your ears."
Upper arms	"Raise your finger tips to your shoulders and tense your biceps."
Lower arms	"Clench your fists tightly."
Back	"Pull your shoulder blades back as if they are trying to meet."
Chest	"Take a deep breath and hold for about 10 seconds."
Abdomen	"Pull in your stomach towards your back."
Hips	"Squeeze the muscles of your rear end."
Thighs	"Press your thighs together tightly."
Lower legs	"Point your toes out."

suggestions to "smooth out," "loosen," "unwind," or "relax" the muscles or simply to "let go of tension." The lower forehead is tensed by drawing the eyebrows down and furrowing the forehead. The eye area is tensed by shutting the eyes tightly (not too tightly if the client is wearing contacts). Tension in the mouth is produced by closing the lips tightly or by pursing the lips. The jaw is tensed by moving the lower jaw forward and pulling the corners of the mouth back. Tension is created at the back of the neck by moving the chin down close to the collar bone. The shoulder area is tensed by bringing the shoulders up toward the ears. The upper arms are tensed by raising the hands toward the same-side shoulders and squeezing the bicep muscles. The lower arms are tensed by closing the fists tightly. The back is tensed by pulling the shoulder blades well back. The chest area is tensed by holding a deep breath for about 10 seconds. The abdomen is tensed by tightening or crunching the stomach muscles. The hip area is tensed by squeezing the gluteus maximus muscles. The thighs are tensed by pressing the knees or thighs together tightly. The lower legs and feet are tensed by pointing the toes down.

At the end of this training, and before the first PMR exercise is initiated, the client should be asked to rate and record his or her anxiety and tension in the "Before-practice rating" section of the Relaxation Diary (see Handout 6.1). As in earlier handouts, anxiety is rated on a 0–8 scale (where 0 means no anxiety and 8 indicates an extreme level of anxiety). Tension is also rated on a 0–8 scale (where 0 indicates deep muscular relaxation or the absence of tension, 2 is mild tension, 4 is moderate tension, 6 is severe tension, and 8 is extreme tension). The client will be asked to make these ratings again after the completion of the first PMR exercise.

Part 2: Implementing the Tension–Release Relaxation Exercise. The therapist can refer to the script contained in Table 6.3 for the in-session tension–release PMR training exercise. The exercise consists of four or five parts: tensing and relaxing muscle groups, deepening the relaxation, positive imagery (optional), focusing on the breath, and ending the exercise. Throughout the exercise, the therapist should read the script in a rhythmic (but relatively monotone) and soothing voice.

When the first in-session relaxation practice is complete, the therapist should ask the client for feedback (e.g., "How was that?"), and again ask the client to rate anxiety and tension on the Relaxation Diary (see Handout 6.1). Every practice is to be recorded on this form. Any difficulties with the exercise should be discussed or noted in the "Comments" section of the form. These difficulties are to be addressed in session. Potential problems with mastering relaxation skills are discussed in the last section of this chapter.

The therapist can give the client the audiotape of the exercise at the end of the first in-session practice and instruct the client to practice the exercise twice a day. During the first week, the first few days of practice are to be done with the tape. On the following days, one practice per day is to be done with the tape, and the second practice from memory of the exercise. The therapist should tell the client that he or she should be able to do the exercise without the tape by the second week of training. If the client has a lot of difficulty completing the exercise without the tape, however, he or she should continue using the tape and should discuss any difficulties with the therapist. Training is sufficient when the client can consistently (i.e., throughout 2 full weeks) lower the after-practice ratings of anxiety and tension to 1 or 0 on the Relaxation Diary with the PMR exercise.

RELAXATION DIARY

Rating scale for anxiety and tension

0	1	2	3	4	5	6	7	8
None		Mild		Moderate		Severe		Extreme

Time	Date	Before-practice ratings anxiety/tension	After-practice ratings anxiety/tension	Comments

TABLE 6.3. Script for Tension–Release 15-Muscle-Group PMR

Introduction

Settle yourself into a comfortable position on a couch, bed, or recliner. Let your body be fully supported and close your eyes gently. Now I want you to listen to my words and to the sound of my voice. Clear your mind of everything else. Let all other sounds fade away.

Part I: Tensing and relaxing the muscle groups

Now I want you to focus your attention on your scalp and upper forehead. Raise your eyebrows up to wrinkle your forehead. Notice the tension in your scalp and upper forehead [*pause for about 5 seconds*].

Now release the tension in your scalp and forehead [*pause*], letting go of all tension and smoothing out the muscles [*pause*]. Notice the sensations of relaxation [*pause for about 10 seconds*].

Now focus your attention on your lower forehead. Pull your eyebrows down into a frown. Notice the tension in your lower forehead [*pause about 5 seconds*].

Now relax the muscles in your lower forehead [*pause*], letting go of all tension and loosening up the muscles [*pause*]. Notice the sensations of relaxation [*pause about 10 seconds*].

Now focus on the area around your eyes. Close your eyes tightly (but not too tightly, if wearing contacts). Notice the tension around your eyes [*pause about 5 seconds*].

Now let go of the tension in your eye area [*pause*], unwinding the muscles [*pause*] and relaxing them completely [*pause*]. If you begin to feel drowsy or sleepy, that is fine; just let yourself become more and more relaxed [*pause about 10 seconds*].

Now focus on the area of your mouth. Purse your lips. Notice the tensions in your mouth area [*pause about 5 seconds*].

Now relax the muscles of your mouth [*pause*], opening up and loosening the muscles [*pause*]. Notice the comfortable sensations as you are becoming more and more relaxed [*pause about 10 seconds*].

Now focus on your jaw area. Push your chin out and pull the corners of your mouth back. Notice the tension in your jaw area [*pause about 5 seconds*].

Now release the tension of your jaw area [*pause*], letting your jaw drop slightly [*pause*], and relaxing all of the muscles [*pause*]. Notice the pleasant sensations as you are relaxing more and more deeply [*pause about 10 seconds*].

Now focus on the area at the back of your neck. Lower your chin until it almost touches your collar bone. Notice the tension at the back of your neck [*pause about 5 seconds*].

Now relax the muscles at the back of your neck [*pause*], unwinding and loosening the muscles [*pause*]. Notice the soothing sensation as you're body is relaxing, further and further [*pause about 10 seconds*].

Now focus on your shoulder area. Raise your shoulders up close to your ears. Notice the tension in your shoulder area [*pause about 5 seconds*].

Now release the tension in your shoulder area [*pause*], letting the muscles become relaxed and limp [*pause*]. Notice the feeling of heaviness as your muscles relax completely [*pause about 10 seconds*].

Now focus on your upper arms. Raise your fingertips to your shoulders and tense your biceps. Notice the tension in your upper arms [*pause about 5 seconds*].

Now let go of the tension in your upper arms [*pause*]; let it all melt away [*pause*]. Notice the feeling of warmth in your body as you become more and more relaxed [*pause about 10 seconds*].

Now focus on your lower arms and hands. Clench your fists tightly. Notice the tension in your hands and lower arms [*pause about 5 seconds*].

Now open your hands [*pause*], release all tension and relax [*pause*]. Notice the comfortable sensation of relaxation as it goes down and farther down throughout your body [*pause about 10 seconds*].

Now focus on the muscles of your back. Pull your shoulder blades back as if they are trying to meet. Notice the tension in your back [*pause about 5 seconds*].

Now relax the muscles in your back [*pause*], letting it round out [*pause*]. Notice the pleasant feelings as you go into a deeper and deeper state of relaxation [*pause about 10 seconds*].

Now focus on your chest area. Take in a deep breath and hold for about 10 seconds. Notice the tension in your chest area [*pause about 5 seconds*].

(continued)

TABLE 6.3. (*continued*)

Now release your breath and relax your chest area [*pause*]. With each breath, feel the relaxation increasing each time you breath in [*pause*] and the relaxation spreading throughout your body as you breath out [*pause about 10 seconds*].

Now focus on your abdomen. Pull your stomach in towards your back. Notice the tension in your abdomen [*pause about 5 seconds*].

Now relax your abdomen [*pause*], loosening the muscle and letting it go [*pause*]. The relaxation is growing deeper and deeper, farther and farther down into every part of your body [*pause about 10 seconds*].

Now focus on your hip area. Tense the muscles of your rear end. Notice the tension in your hip area [*pause about 5 seconds*].

Now relax the muscles of your hip area [*pause*]. Feel yourself sinking deep into the chair [*pause*]; you are going deeper and deeper into a deep state of relaxation [*pause for 10 seconds*].

Now focus on your thigh area. Press your thighs together tightly. Notice the tension in your thigh area [*pause about 5 seconds*].

Now relax the muscles of your thigh area [*pause*], unwinding and loosening every part of your body [*pause*]. Feel calm and quiet as your body and mind relax completely [*pause about 10 seconds*].

Now focus on your lower legs and feet. Point your toes outward. Notice the tension in your lower legs and feet [*pause about 5 seconds*].

Now relax the muscles of your lower legs and feet [*pause*], letting go and loosening up [*pause*]. Notice the very restful and very peaceful feelings of deep relaxation throughout every part of your body [*pause about 10 seconds*].

Part II: Intensifying the relaxation

Now I want you to continue relaxing all of the muscles of your body: your forehead and face, your neck and shoulder area, your back and chest, your abdomen and hip area, your arms and legs. Let all your muscles become more and more deeply relaxed. I'm going to help you enter a deeper state of relaxation by counting from one to five. As I begin counting, you will feel yourself going farther and farther down into a very deep state of relaxation [*pause*]. One [*pause*], you are becoming more deeply relaxed. Two [*pause*], down, down into a deeply restful state. Three [*pause*], farther and farther down into a very relaxed state. Four [*pause*], more and more deeply relaxed. Five [*pause*], deeply relaxed [*pause about 10 seconds*].

Part III: Positive imagery (optional)

The following script may be used, but only if the client experiences this scenario as one in which he or she feels calm, peaceful, and relaxed. Other, more individualized, scripts may be developed by the therapist and client. In developing such scripts, the therapist and client should describe the scenario through all five senses. The client's primary sense modality should be emphasized throughout. The script becomes more effective the more vivid the descriptions.

Now I want you to imagine that you are lying on a beach. It's one of those long, hot, lazy summer days. Overhead, you see the bright blue sky and the warm yellow sun. You gently close your eyes and feel the strong warm rays of the sun. Your body soaks up the warmth [*pause*]. The sand underneath is soft. It molds to your body and cradles you [*pause*]. A gentle cool breeze wafts over the water. It is welcome relief from the steady warmth of the sun [*pause*]. The ocean air leaves a salty taste on your lips [*pause*]. As you lay, you hear the calling of the gulls above. You hear the gentle and rhythmic sound of the waves. As the waves rush in and the waves rush out, your mind is being rocked into a very restful state. You feel soothed and at complete peace [*pause about 10 seconds*].

Part IV: Focusing on the breath

Now I want you to remain in this very relaxed and restful state. I want you to attend to your breathing. Notice the coolness of the air as it enters your nostrils [*try to pair statement with inhalation and then pause*]. Notice the air passing slowly and deeply down, expanding your diaphragm [*pause*]. And notice

(continued)

TABLE 6.3. (continued)

the warmth and moisture of the air as it slowly passes back out through your nose [*try to pair statement with exhalation and then pause*]. Just continue to attend to your breathing and to these sensations [*pause*]. Now each time you inhale, mentally say "re" and each time you exhale, mentally say "lax." [*Pairing with inhalations and exhalations:*] Inhale "re", exhale "lax." [*Repeat several times.*]

Part V: Ending the exercise

Now I am going to help you arise from this very deep state of relaxation to a state of complete alertness. Shortly, I will start counting backwards from five to one. As I count, you will feel yourself gradually becoming more and more alert, more and more refreshed. When I reach the count of two, I want you to open your eyes. On the count of one, you will feel as if you have just fully awoken from a rejuvenating nap [*pause*]. Ready? Five [*pause*], you are beginning to become more alert. Four [*pause*], you feel yourself coming up into a more alert state. Three [*pause*], more and more alert. Two [*pause*], your eyes are now open and you are feeling very refreshed. One [*pause*], you are now feeling fully alert and fully refreshed.

From *Treating Generalized Anxiety Disorder* by Jayne L. Rygh and William C. Sanderson. Copyright 2004 by The Guilford Press. Permission to photocopy this table is granted to purchasers of this book for personal use only (see copyright page for details).

Step 2: The Relaxation-Only PMR Exercise

This version of the PMR exercise is identical to the one just described except that the script for Part I is altered. This new script (see Table 6.4) eliminates the tensing of muscles and instructs the client to release existing tension and relax. All other parts of the exercise are exactly the same. The benefit of mastering this version of the exercise is that it can be practiced without others noticing. The client can use this exercise as a tool to intentionally relax his or her body anywhere.

The same environmental conditions should be created for initial practices. An audiotape of this version is not created for the client. Practices ideally should be done twice a day, but once is sufficient. When the client's after-practice ratings of anxiety and tension are consistently 1 or 0 on the Relaxation Diary for this exercise, the client can begin practices under more stimulating and distracting conditions. For example, the client can practice while sitting on the subway or train to work and, later, practice the exercise while watching a TV program. The conditions for practices can increasingly approach those of normal daily life.

An Alternative Version of PMR

Wolpe (1958) developed another version of PMR. Öst (1987) utilized this version in his AR technique, to be described later in this chapter. This alternative version of PMR has three phases, each lasting 1–2 weeks. An overview of this version as described by Öst (1987) is provided in Table 6.5.

The first phase of training is usually completed in two weekly sessions. All exercises in this phase are carried out in an upright position in a comfortable chair with eyes closed. The between-session assignment is for twice-a-day practice, with each practice recorded on the Relaxation Diary. The client is not given a tape with this training.

TABLE 6.4. Replacement Script for Part I: Relaxing the Muscle Groups

Part I: Relaxing the muscle groups

Now I want you to focus your attention on your scalp and upper forehead and release any tension [*pause*], smoothing out and relaxing the muscles [*pause*]. Notice the sensations of relaxation [*pause for about 10 seconds*].

Now focus your attention on your lower forehead and relax the muscles [*pause*], letting go and loosening up the muscles [*pause*]. Notice the sensations of relaxation [*pause about 10 seconds*].

Now focus on the area around your eyes and let go of any tension [*pause*], unwinding the muscles [*pause*] and relaxing them completely [*pause*]. If you begin to feel drowsy or sleepy, that is fine; just let yourself become more and more relaxed [*pause about 10 seconds*].

Now focus on the area of your mouth and relax the muscles [*pause*], opening up and loosening the muscles [*pause*]. Notice the comfortable sensations as you are becoming more and more relaxed [*pause about 10 seconds*].

Now focus on your jaw area and release any tension [*pause*], letting your jaw drop slightly [*pause*], and relaxing all of the muscles [*pause*]. Notice the pleasant sensations as you are relaxing more and more deeply [*pause about 10 seconds*].

Now focus on the area at the back of your neck and relax the muscles [*pause*], unwinding and loosening the muscles [*pause*]. Notice the soothing sensation as your body is relaxing, further and further [*pause about 10 seconds*].

Now focus on your shoulder area and release any tension [*pause*], letting the muscles become relaxed and limp [*pause*]. Notice the feeling of heaviness as your muscles relax completely [*pause about 10 seconds*].

Now focus on your upper arms and let go of any tension [*pause*]; let it all melt away [*pause*]. Notice the feeling of warmth in your body as you become more and more relaxed [*pause about 10 seconds*].

Now focus on your lower arms and hands and release any tension [*pause*], letting go and releasing [*pause*]. Notice the comfortable sensation of relaxation as it is goes down and farther down throughout your body [*pause about 10 seconds*].

Now focus on the muscles of your back and relax the muscles [*pause*], letting it round out [*pause*]. Notice the pleasant feelings as you go into a deeper and deeper state of relaxation [*pause about 10 seconds*].

Now focus on your chest area and relax this area [*pause*]. With each breath, feel relaxation increasing each time you breath in [*pause*] and relaxation spreading throughout your body as you breath out [*pause about 10 seconds*].

Now focus on your abdomen and release any tension [*pause*], loosening and letting go [*pause*]. The relaxation is growing deeper and deeper, farther and farther down into every part of your body [*pause about 10 seconds*].

Now focus on your hip area and relax the muscles [*pause*]. Feel yourself sinking deep into the chair [*pause*]; you are going deeper and deeper into a deep state of relaxation [*pause for 10 seconds*].

Now focus on your thigh area and on letting go of any tension [*pause*], unwinding and loosening every part of your body [*pause*]. Feel calm and quiet as your body and mind relax completely [*pause about 10 seconds*].

Now focus on your lower legs and feet and relax the muscles [*pause*], letting go and loosening up [*pause*]. Notice the very restful and very peaceful feelings of deep relaxation throughout every part of your body [*pause about 10 seconds*].

TABLE 6.5. Overview of Alternative PMR

Phase I. Tense and release (two weekly sessions)

Session 1: Read basic script (see Table 6.3) for tensing and releasing each of the following upper body muscle groups: (1) both hands, (2) both arms, (3) face, (4) neck, and (5) both shoulders. For each group, tense for 5 seconds; relax for 15 seconds.

Session 2: To the upper-body groups above, add the following lower-body groups: (6) back, (7) chest, (8) stomach, (9) hips, (10) both legs, and (11) both feet. For each group, tense for 5 seconds; relax for 15 seconds. (Allow 15–20 minutes for entire exercise)

Phase II. Release only (one or two weekly sessions)

Session 3–4: Release only for all muscle groups in Session 2. Use the following script (allow 5–10 minutes for entire exercise):

"Breathe with calm, regular breaths and feel how you relax more and more for every breath. . . . Just let go. . . . Relax your forehead . . . eyebrows . . . eyelids . . . jaws . . . tongue and throat . . . lips . . . your entire face. . . . Relax your neck . . . shoulders . . . arms . . . hands . . . and all the way out to your fingertips. . . . Breathe calmly and regularly with your stomach all the time. . . . Let the relaxation spread to your stomach . . . waist and back. . . . Relax the lower part of your body, your behind . . . thighs . . . knees . . . calves . . . feet . . . and all the way down to the tips of your toes. . . . Breathe calmly and regularly and feel how you relax more and more by each breath. . . . Take a deep breath and hold your breath for a couple of seconds . . . and let the air out slowly . . . slowly. . . . Notice how you relax more and more."

Phase III. Cue-controlled relaxation (one or two weekly sessions)

Sessions 4–6: Begin with release-only exercise. When client is deeply relaxed, says "inhale" cued to client's inhalations and "relax" just before exhalation. Repeat five times. Client then is instructed to mentally repeat "inhale" and "relax" with each inhalation and exhalation, to achieve a deep state of relaxation without therapist assistance. Repeat four or five times. Client is then asked to estimate time to achieve relaxed state with this last method. Inaccurate estimates are corrected. Most clients achieve deep relaxation in 2–3 minutes.

Note. The Phase II script is reprinted from, and the rest of the table is adapted from, Öst (1987, Appendix A). Copyright 1987 by Elsevier. Reprinted/adapted by permission.

The first of these sessions trains the client in how to tense and release tension in major muscle groups of the upper body: both hands, both arms, face, neck, and both shoulders. The relaxation exercise is carried out with these muscle groups only. Tension is held for 5 seconds and relaxation is held for 15 seconds in each muscle group. The major muscle groups of the lower part of the body—back, chest, stomach, hips, both legs, and both feet—are added to the exercise in the second session. The entire exercise should take between 15 and 20 minutes. The therapist can modify the PMR script in Table 6.3 for these exercises (see the preceding section for general instructions on applications).

The second phase is usually is completed in 1–2 weekly sessions. The relaxation exercise is altered by eliminating the tensing portion of the exercise and using a release-only version. If any tension is experienced in a particular muscle group during this version of the exercise, that muscle group should be briefly tensed and then relaxed. This exercise should take 5–10 minutes to complete. Öst has provided a script for the release-only phase (see Table 6.5).

The third phase is cue-controlled relaxation and usually takes 1–2 weeks of training. During this phase, the word "relax" is conditioned to evoke a deep state of relaxation. The focus is on the breathing in this stage. The sessions begin with the release-only exercise. Once the client is deeply relaxed, the client signals the therapist by raising an index finger. The therapist then gives the following instructions, cued to the client's breathing: "inhale"during inhalation and "relax" right before the client exhales. This is repeated five times. The client then is instructed to mentally repeat the same words during the breathing cycle for about 1 minute. (The word "relax" can be used in isolation, if this is preferred.) The client is then instructed to estimate the time he or she needs to achieve a deeply relaxed state with each exercise. If estimates are inaccurate they are corrected. Most clients are able to achieve deep relaxation within 2–3 minutes with this exercise.

DIAPHRAGMATIC BREATHING

Similar to PMR, DB is a skill that can increase the client's control over physiological processes. DB gives the client a simple tool for quickly calming the body. This technique was introduced by Clark, Salkovskis, and Chalkley (1985) for panic disorder. The therapist can educate the client with the fact that DB has been shown to be helpful for a variety of symptoms (e.g., headaches, high blood pressure, insomnia, hyperventilation, Raynaud's syndrome), in addition to anxiety. Like PMR, DB is a skill that can only be mastered with regular practice. An overview of the DB technique is presented in Table 6.6.

TABLE 6.6. Overview of Diaphragmatic Breathing (DB) Technique

1. Offer basic information on breathing.
   • Lungs do not have any muscles of their own.
   • The diaphragm controls size and frequency of breaths.
   • Breathing is primarily automatic, but can be controlled to some extent through the diaphragm.
   • The diaphragm contracts when a person is stressed; breathing turns shallow and rapid; upper chest and shoulders rise up and down with breaths.
   • When relaxed, diaphragm muscles are loose; breathing slows, deepens; abdomen rises and falls with breaths.
   • The purpose of DB is to breathe voluntarily as if the body is in a relaxed state.
2. Client should loosen any tight clothing around waist and abdomen.
3. Client places one hand on the chest and the other on the abdomen.
4. Observe movements of client's hands; in DB, only the hand on the abdomen moves, while the hand on the chest is still.
5. If DB is not yet achieved, tell client to relax abdomen muscles, to expand abdomen during inhalations, and to keep the chest area still.
6. Once the correct pattern of breathing is mastered, have client slow pace to 8–10 breathing cycles per minute.
7. When the pattern and pace of breathing are mastered, have client mentally focus on the word "relax." Client should mentally say "re" with each inhalation, "lax" with each exhalation.
8. Client should let other thoughts and images go, and focus attention on the word "relax" and the sensations of muscular relaxation.

Note. Based on Clark, Salkoviskis, and Chalkley (1985).

The therapist may want to start the first training session by presenting some basic information about breathing. For the most part, breathing is an automatic process, controlled by sensors in the lungs that communicate with the brain. The muscle that controls the size and frequency of the breaths is the diaphragm. The lungs do not contain any muscles of their own. When an individual is anxious or stressed, the diaphragm automatically constricts. Breathing becomes more shallow and rapid. In addition, the individual may attempt to catch his or her breath by taking in large, shallow breaths. One can observe the upper chest moving in and out and the shoulders rising up and down when an individual is anxious or stressed. When an individual is relaxed, the diaphragm is loose. Breathing automatically slows and is deeper. Air is taken into the diaphragmatic area of the body. It appears as if the person is breathing through his or her abdomen when relaxed. Although the functioning of the diaphragm muscle is largely an automatic process, this process can be brought under some degree of voluntary control. The purpose of DB is to breathe consciously and purposefully as if the body is in a relaxed state. This change in the pattern of breathing can alter the body's processes toward those that occur naturally in a relaxed state.

Before beginning training in DB, the therapist should check whether the client has learned this skill in other settings (e.g., voice lessons, yoga, etc.). If so, the therapist may want to check that it is being done correctly, and then therapist and client can skip to the meditation component of the exercise. If not, the therapist will need to train the client.

To start with, any tight clothing around the client's waist and abdomen should be loosened. A variety of positions can be used to practice: sitting in a comfortable and relaxed position; standing up and bending slightly forward at the waist; or lying on one's back on a bed, in the floor, or in a recliner. In the initial phase of training, the client may want to experiment with different positions to find what works best. Once in position, the client is instructed to place one hand on the chest and the other hand on the abdomen. The hand on the abdomen should be placed so that the navel is between the ring finger and pinky finger.

Both the therapist and client can observe the client's breathing by watching the movement of the client's hands. Depending upon the pattern of breathing, it can be used as an example. In DB, only the hand on the diaphragm moves; the shoulders and chest under the other hand should be still.

If necessary, the therapist should demonstrate the correct pattern of breathing for the client, and then instruct the client to relax the muscles of the abdomen. The therapist can ask the client to expand the abdomen during inhalations, and to try to hold the chest area still. The therapist may suggest that the client think of the abdomen as a balloon filling and emptying with air. The therapist can then mirror any problems demonstrated by the client and repeat the demonstration of the correct breathing pattern. The therapist can also suggest that the client check his or her breathing in front of a mirror during practices at home. Once the client demonstrates control of the breathing, the client can be instructed to slow the pace of breathing to 8–10 cycles per minute.

After these mechanical aspects of the skill are mastered, the client can begin to incorporate the meditation component of the exercise. This involves having the client focus internally on the word "relax." The purpose of this is to increase control over the focus of attention. The meditation component helps counter distractibility during episodes of excessive worry.

With each inhalation, the client should mentally say "re"; with each exhalation, he or she should say "lax." Each time the client repeats the word "re-lax," the client should let all muscles become as loose, heavy, and relaxed as possible. If other thoughts or images are noticed, the client is to let them go. Attention should be repeatedly refocused on the word "relax," and the feelings of muscular relaxation.

Practice is essential in order to gain mastery of the skill of DB. The therapist should instruct the client to practice diaphragmatic DB multiple times throughout the day. Lack of practice may prevent mastery of this skill.

SELF-CONTROL DESENSITIZATION

The S-CD technique, developed by Goldfried (1971), is an outgrowth of Wolpe's (1958) systematic desensitization technique. Systematic desensitization is based on the notion that tension and relaxation responses are mutually exclusive. It consists of graded exposures to anxiety-provoking stimuli via imagery, within the context of a deep relaxation exercise. Its purpose is to increase the client's control over worry by providing a coping technique for interrupting the spiraling process of anxiety and worry. The technique teaches the client how to catch this spiral early and to intervene with relaxation. Theoretically, the repeated pairing of anxiety-provoking stimuli with a deep relaxation response strengthens the associations between such stimuli and this response.

The specific application of S-CD for GAD (Borkovec et al., 1987) involves presenting particular worries within the context of a deep relaxation exercise. Ideally, the cognitive, physiological, and behavioral urges associated with each worry are activated along with the worry itself during this exercise. When increases in anxiety are noticed, clients are instructed to return to a deeply relaxed state.

Prior to implementation of this technique, clients must have mastered obtaining a deep state of relaxation through PMR or DB. Positive imagery alone (or, more specifically, positive coping imagery) may also be used if a deep state of relaxation can be achieved through this method. An overview of the S-CD technique is presented in Table 6.7.

Prior to introducing this technique, the therapist should review the client's completed Worry Episode Logs (for Treatment) and session notes to facilitate the in-session process of identifying specific worries for a hierarchy of worries (see Handout 6.2). The therapist begins the first session with this technique by explaining its purpose and the general procedure. A hierarchy of worries is then developed with the client.

Different episodes of worry with different intensity levels of anxiety must be identified. The episode's triggers and worry responses should be rated on the usual 0–8 scale (with 0 representing no anxiety and 8 extreme anxiety). The triggers are then arranged in a hierarchy from the least to the most anxiety-provoking. Richard's hierarchy is provided in Figure 6.1.

Items for the S-CD exercises are selected from this hierarchy of worries. For the first practice, a very low-level item from this hierarchy is selected. The client is then asked to provide detailed information about any images, thoughts, assumptions, and/or beliefs; physiological activities; and behavioral urges associated with that item. The therapist creates a rough script that incorporates this information for the exercise. This script is used during the S-CD exercise to facilitate provocation of worry. During the exercises, the client is instructed to raise an index finger to signal increased anxiety and to lower the finger when he or she is deeply relaxed.

TABLE 6.7. Overview of Self-Control Desensitization (S-CD) Technique

1. Review Completed Worry Episode Logs (for Treatment) and notes to gather possible items for the hierarchy before the session introducing the technique to the client.

2. Introduce the technique to the client, and develop a hierarchy of worry triggers and responses drawn from the worry episodes (see Handout 6.2).

3. A low-ranking trigger is selected first.

4. Collect detailed information from the client about cognitions, physiological arousal, and behavioral urges related to this item. Then create a rough script that can be flexibly used to evoke worry during the exercise.

5. The desensitization exercise itself begins with the client deeply relaxing and lowering an index finger to indicate a relaxed state.

6. Narrate the script of the worrisome event.

7. The client raises an index finger to indicate increased anxiety during the narration of the script.

8. Remind the client to return to a deeply relaxed state with relaxation skills or positive coping imagery (see Chapter 5). When the client's index finger is again lowered, the narration continues.

9. Exercise is repeated for the same item until the client can relax within 7 seconds or is able to hold a relaxed state during the narration for a least 1 minute on three occasions.

10. A new, more anxiety-provoking item is then selected from the hierarchy, and Steps 4–8 are repeated.

Note. Based on Goldfried (1971).

From *Treating Generalized Anxiety Disorder* by Jayne L. Rygh and William C. Sanderson. Copyright 2004 by The Guilford Press. Permission to photocopy this table is granted to purchasers of this book for personal use only (see copyright page for details).

The exercise begins with the client purposefully entering a deep state of relaxation. When the client lowers his or her index finger, the therapist begins to narrate the script of the anxiety-provoking event. If the client raises his or her index finger at any point in the narration, the therapist reminds the client to return purposefully to a deep state of relaxation while continuing to focus attention on the scripted imagery, if possible. When the client has successfully returned to a deep state of relaxation, the narration continues. The therapist repeats the exercise with the worry trigger until the client is able to relax fairly quickly (within 7 seconds) or is able to hold a deeply relaxed state for at least 1 minute.

The following clinical vignette illustrates the application of the S-CD technique with the lowest-level item on Richard's hierarchy of worries (see Figure 6.1).

THERAPIST: Now I want you to deeply relax yourself. . . .

CLIENT: (*After a pause, client signals by lowering index finger.*)

THERAPIST: Imagine you're at the ice rink with your daughter. Make the image as real as possible for yourself . . . feel the cold air against your face, the slippery and hard ice underfoot, see the crowd of people skating around the rink. . . . Hear the music. . . . Involve all of your senses. . . . Imagine yourself with your daughter skating. . . . You are holding hands. . . . Her little hand feels small and fragile.

CLIENT: (*After about a minute, the client raises finger.*)

THERAPIST: Stay with the image, and counter these feelings with deep relaxation. Just let yourself become deeply relaxed. . . .

HIERARCHY OF WORRIES FORM

Worry trigger: _____ Anxiety level (0–8): ____
    Physical response: _____
    Cognitive response: _____
    Behavioral response: _____

Worry trigger: _____ Anxiety level (0–8): ____
    Physical response: _____
    Cognitive response: _____
    Behavioral response: _____

Worry trigger: _____ Anxiety level (0–8): ____
    Physical response: _____
    Cognitive response: _____
    Behavioral response: _____

Worry trigger: _____ Anxiety level (0–8): ____
    Physical response: _____
    Cognitive response: _____
    Behavioral response: _____

Worry trigger: _____ Anxiety level (0–8): ____
    Physical response: _____
    Cognitive response: _____
    Behavioral response: _____

Worry trigger: _____ Anxiety level (0–8): ____
    Physical response: _____
    Cognitive response: _____
    Behavioral response: _____

Worry trigger: _____ Anxiety level (0–8): ____
    Physical response: _____
    Cognitive response: _____
    Behavioral response: _____

Worry trigger: _____ Anxiety level (0–8): ____
    Physical response: _____
    Cognitive response: _____
    Behavioral response: _____

HIERARCHY OF WORRIES FORM

Worry trigger: Skating with daughter at the ice rink.   Anxiety level (0–8): 2
    Physical response: Tension in face and shoulders.
    Cognitive response: A kid might run into her. What if she breaks a bone?
    Behavioral response: Skate behind her. Watch her and other kids closely.

Worry trigger: A minor error in a brief sent to boss.   Anxiety level (0–8): 3
    Physical response: Tension in facial, neck, and shoulder areas.
    Cognitive response: I'm a jerk not to have checked. My boss will be unhappy.
    Behavioral response: Continue to review brief for other errors.

Worry trigger: Colleague gets honorable mention from judge.   Anxiety level (0–8): 4
    Physical response: Tension in chest, shoulder, and neck area.
    Cognitive response: I've done nothing of special note. I'm not succeeding.
    Behavioral response: I stay very late at work and take on new assignments.

Worry trigger: Stuck in subway tunnel on way to a new client.   Anxiety level (0–8): 5
    Physical response: Shallow breathing. Tension in arms, legs, and neck.
    Cognitive response: Image of client looking furious and firing our firm.
    Behavioral response: Look at watch every few seconds. Stand up repeatedly.

Worry trigger: A toilet at home starts to leak.   Anxiety level (0–8): 6
    Physical response: Tension in shoulder and leg areas.
    Cognitive response: Image of major plumbing problems. We'll be broke.
    Behavioral response: Pacing and calculating worst-case scenarios.

Worry trigger: Image of being humiliated by a judge in court.   Anxiety level (0–8): 7
    Physical response: Shallow breath, heart pounding, tension in face and chest.
    Cognitive response: I'll be sanctioned. The firm will be sued. I'll be ruined.
    Behavioral response: Repeatedly rehearse next day's appearance in court.

Worry trigger: Partner's daughter died from a serious illness.   Anxiety level (0–8): 8
    Physical response: Rapid heartbeat, chest breathing, overall body tension.
    Cognitive response: Image of my own kid's funeral. I can't handle this.
    Behavioral response: Checked on kids and observed kids for illness repeatedly.

Worry trigger: Image of client complaining to boss about me.   Anxiety level (0–8): 8
    Physical response: Extreme tension in facial, neck, and shoulder areas.
    Cognitive response: I'll be fired. Image of self as homeless.
    Behavioral response: Checked want ads. Checking family savings repeatedly.

FIGURE 6.1. Richard's Hierarchy of Worries Form.

CLIENT: (*After about a minute, the client lowers finger.*)

THERAPIST: Notice the teenagers skating. Hear how noisy they are. You see them darting about and skating quickly between other people.

CLIENT: (*After a few seconds, client raises finger and opens his eyes.*)

THERAPIST: Close your eyes and tell me what's happening in the image.

CLIENT: A teenager has cut between us, and my daughter has fallen on the ice. She's crying . . . I'm tense. I'm worried she's hurt.

THERAPIST: Stay with the image, and counter these feelings with deep relaxation.

CLIENT: I can't. I see her mouth bleeding. . . . I'm really tense. I can't stand this image! I want to stop this exercise.

THERAPIST: Hold on to the image. Try to stick with the image. Remember that I am here to help you cope. Remind yourself that this is just an image, a frightening image, and nothing else.

CLIENT: OK.

THERAPIST: Now focus on your daughter's mouth and see a tiny little cut of no significance. . . . Now, locate the areas of tension in your body. . . . Now relax those areas. Release the tension. . . . Just let the tension in your muscles go as you become more deeply relaxed . . . loose, heavy, and relaxed. . . . Continue focusing on calming yourself. Breathe slowly and regularly through your nose. Mentally repeat the word "relax" each time you exhale. Breathe slowly and deeply through your diaphragm. . . . Tell me what is happening now.

CLIENT: (*Pause*) . . . I see it's a little cut . . . not serious. I tell her and myself to relax, that the pain will pass. . . . (*Client is practicing the relaxation exercise again. He lowers his finger after a couple of minutes pass.*)

THERAPIST: Continue to relax all of your muscles. Let your body be as loose and relaxed as possible as you glide around the rink with your daughter. . . . Picture yourself chatting and smiling with your daughter as you glide around the ice. Continue to hold on to those images. Signal if any anxiety returns.

In the example above, Richard jumps to an image associated with a much higher level of anxiety in the middle of the exercise. If this occurs, the therapist should strongly encourage the client to stick with the more anxiety-provoking image (or other trigger) and give reassurance that the therapist will actively assist the client with coping. If possible, the therapist can then attempt to refocus the client's attention on the lower-level anxiety item. If this occurs during practices between sessions, or if the client insists on terminating the exercise with the therapist, it is important to permit the client to terminate the exercise. In these instances, the therapist should have the client rate the level of anxiety associated with that exercise. The therapist can frame the experience as one in which the level of anxiety is too high, and the client's desire to avoid is overpowering the desire to approach and attempt to cope. If the client interprets stopping the exercise as a personal failure or a failure of the technique, the therapist can reframe the experience as something that naturally occurs when there has not yet been sufficient opportunity to develop the necessary coping skills for dealing with higher levels of anxiety. The therapist should tell the client that it is acceptable to terminate the exercise in such instances and to refocus on relaxation only. When problems occur with between-session practices, the client should note problems so that they can be dealt with in future sessions.

Particular worry scenarios should be repeated until the client has been able to successfully counter worry with deep relaxation on at least three occasions. The goal is for the client to maintain a relaxed state for at least 60 seconds or to lower the anxiety responses significantly within 7 seconds over a minimum of three occasions of imaging a particular scenario. If the client experiences difficulties in lowering his or her anxiety by the end of a 60-second period, the client should be instructed to stop imaging that particular worry scenario and to return to the deep relaxation exercise for approximately 60 seconds. The client may need to elicit and practice coping with one aspect of worry at a time (e.g., specific attributes of an image) before proceeding to other aspects of the worry (e.g., other attributes of an image plus the meaning associated with that image). The same scene should be repeated until the client achieves success, as noted above. The client should progress to items on the hierarchy associated with higher levels of anxiety only after he or she has mastered the lower-level items.

APPLIED RELAXATION

The goal of AR is to demonstrate relaxation as an effective coping strategy for significantly reducing anxiety under many circumstances (Borkovec & Costello, 1993). AR is similar to the S-CD technique in that relaxation is applied to anxiety-provoking stimuli. The difference between the two techniques is that AR is practiced across a large range of anxiety-rousing situations in daily life, rather than imaginally. The most thoroughly researched method of AR in the treatment of GAD was developed by Öst (1987).

The steps for implementing the AR technique are presented in Table 6.8. In the first session where this technique is presented, the client identifies situations that elicit arousal and anxiety or worry. Early signs of arousal and anxiety or worry in these situations are identified as cues for applying relaxation. Then the three phases of the alternative PMR training typically occur over the next four to six sessions (see "An Alternative Version of PMR," above). The first phase consists of PMR with tension–release cycles of muscle groups. The second phase consists of PMR with only release of muscle groups. The third phase is cue-controlled relaxation.

The AR technique then proceeds with the practice of cue-controlled relaxation across a wide variety of anxiety-rousing situations in the client's daily life. The client conducts these practices both within therapy sessions and on his or her own between weekly sessions over the next 7–8 weeks. AR is practiced any time arousal and worry are anticipated or noticed.

The therapist instructs the client to relax deeply before entering any situation that typically triggers worry. When any symptoms associated with a worry episode are noticed, the client is to apply the exercise to counteract tension and prevent anxiety from spiraling. The exercise is applied during brief (10- to 15-minute) exposures to anxiety-arousing situations. The client is forewarned that although anxiety reduction may be minimal during initial exposures, the relaxation will increase with repeated practice.

TABLE 6.8. Steps in Implementing Applied Relaxation (AR)

Session 1: Introduction of technique and identification of triggers as cues for AR.

Session 2: Phase I of alternative version of PMR (see Table 6.5).

Session 3: Phase I of alternative version of PMR.

Session 4–5: Phase II of alternative version of PMR.

Session 5–7: Phase III of alternative version of PMR.

Sessions 6–13: In-session and between-session applications of AR.

Sessions 7–19 (biweekly, then monthly as needed): Maintenance and relapse prevention.

Note. Based on Öst (1987).

The final step in the technique is maintenance. The last five or six sessions are spaced biweekly and then monthly, as needed. During this period of treatment, clients are instructed to scan their bodies at least once a day for signs of tension. If tension is noticed at any time throughout a day, cue-controlled relaxation is applied to rid the body of tension. In addition, the clients are to practice cue-controlled relaxation twice a week on a regular basis. Setbacks are predicted and viewed as opportunities to resume practice.

PROBLEMATIC CLIENT RESPONSES TO RELAXATION TECHNIQUES

There are two problems that occasionally arise with relaxation techniques. One is that the client has tried relaxation before, found it ineffective, and is reluctant to try the exercises, again. The other is that the exercises result in increased anxiety and tension.

When prior experiences with relaxation have been ineffective, it is important for the therapist to examine carefully those experiences. The therapist should assess the frequency and duration of practices, and should also determine how well the client was able to focus attention on the exercises. Usually, insufficient or nonsystematic practice of the exercises is responsible for the difficulties. When problems have been due to difficulties with maintaining attention, the therapist can inform the client that such difficulties are relatively common in individuals with GAD. Worries often function as intrusive distractions while clients are practicing the exercises. The therapist can reframe distracting worries as opportunities to practice exerting control over one's focus of attention. When a worry intrudes, permission is given to notice the worry. After noticing the worry, the client should practice letting go of the worry and refocusing attention on the physical sensations experienced during the exercise. The intentional refocusing of attention on stimuli within the moment is a form of mindfulness. (Mindfulness is a technique that will be discussed in Chapter 8.) With repeated practice, the client should find it easier to maintain his or her attention on the exercise. If not, the therapist may want to focus on developing mindfulness skills and return to relaxation training at a later point in treatment.

In cases where the exercise induces anxiety and tension, the therapist should carefully assess the thoughts and images that occur during the exercise, as well as the meaning of relaxation in general for the client. In some instances, the changes in sensations and alertness experienced during the exercise are associated with a loss of control or danger and threat. In other instances, the client may view relaxation as an inefficient use or waste of time, or as overly self-indulgent.

In instances associated with a loss of control or danger and threat, the therapist can alter the relaxation procedure to expose the client more slowly to the feared aspects. Essentially, the relaxation procedure is treated like an exposure exercise. For example, the client can start with only a few muscle groups or practice for shorter periods of time and gradually work up to the full amount.

Clients who either have experienced panic attacks during episodes of worry or have full-blown panic disorder coexisting with their GAD are often frightened by their physical sensations. These clients often fear a loss of control with any change in sensations (e.g., "Something is wrong with my heart"). In such instances, the therapist can provide the following explanation of the changes in sensations experienced during the exercises:

> "As you are practicing this exercise, you are purposely causing physiological changes. These changes are normal and natural alterations of your body's processes. Although you may experience the sensations as unpleasant, they are not at all dangerous. Your heart and respiration rates are decreasing; your gastrointestinal and circulatory systems are slowing; your muscles are releasing tension. During the exercise, you may notice a change in the way your heart is beating. You may notice tingling sensations in your extremities. You may experience muscle twitching. There are a variety of physical sensations that you may notice during this exercise. These sensations are signs that the exercise is working. They are signals that your bodily processes are slowing and that your body is going into a more relaxed state."

When clients believe that relaxation is an inefficient use or a waste of time, the therapist can use an analogy of a reservoir that doesn't receive sufficient rain. Relaxation is like rain. Relaxation replenishes the body's and mind's reservoir of energy. When people allow their bodies and minds to relax, they actually have more energy and become more efficient and productive in the long run. When they deprive themselves of relaxation, their bodies and minds are quickly drained of energy and become less efficient overall.

When clients believe that relaxation is too self-indulgent, they often avoid the exercise to avoid feeling guilty. Often they believe that taking care of others should take precedence over taking care of themselves. The therapist can ask such a client what advice the client would give a friend if the friend neglected taking care of him- or herself in this way. The client's response usually indicates recognition of the problem. It is important to iterate that it is just as important to care for oneself as it is to care for others. When there is a consistent lack of balance in care, it demonstrates a lack of respect for oneself. It can also demonstrate a lack of respect for another when incorrect assumptions are made that the other cannot care for him- or herself. Sitting through the guilt and continuing with the exercises will correct this imbalance. In time, the value of taking care of oneself will become obvious and reinforcing in and of itself.

CHAPTER SEVEN

Treating the Behavioral Component

There are two main goals in treating the behavioral component of GAD: to increase engagement in pleasurable activities, and to decrease excessive and/or unnecessary coping behaviors. In this chapter, we discuss the techniques that target the behavioral component: (1) behavioral response prevention, (2) *in vivo* exposure, and (3) pleasurable activity scheduling.

Deficits in planning, scheduling, and executing pleasurable activities are often apparent in individuals with GAD. The dearth of alternatives for attention and action can intensify difficulties with controlling worry. The technique of pleasurable activity scheduling is used to counteract these deficits by providing adaptive alternatives. We discuss this technique at the end of this chapter.

Although the cognitive restructuring (CR) exercises described in Chapter 5 help the client to recognize the lack of rational support for a specific behavior, the client will continue to experience the urge to act or avoid. Negative reinforcement has conditioned the client not only to think, but also to physically feel, that these coping behaviors are necessary to reduce negative affect and/or experience. This urge is often expressed as reluctance to let go of certain behaviors. One of the therapist's tasks is to help the client understand and break through this reluctance.

As noted in earlier chapters, unnecessary and excessive coping behaviors can take the form of fight, flight, or freeze. Fight behaviors are attempts to counter or overcome threat through aggressive action; flight behaviors are attempts to get away from threat through evasive action; and freeze behaviors are attempts to stop or deter threat by inhibiting action. Fight behaviors can include overpreparation, checking (Schut, Castonguay, & Borkovec, 2001), and overprotection. Flight behaviors can include avoidance, procrastination, evasion, and escape. Freeze behaviors can include stammered speech or halted behaviors. Reassurance seeking—that is, excessive requests for support assistance, or advice—can be either a fight or a flight behavior. It is fight when the purpose is excessive checking; it is flight when the purpose is to flee to a protective figure.

Both fight and flight behaviors may temporarily reduce a client's anxiety, but they also can prevent the client from learning whether or not his or her interpretations of threat are accurate. Although clients may recognize some of their coping behaviors as excessive or unnecessary, they usually have a long history of negative reinforcement that has confirmed, maintained, and strengthened these behaviors. Because individuals with GAD rarely confront the stimuli that evoke worry without executing some coping behaviors, they lack concrete data regarding the actual effectiveness of these behaviors. Response prevention and *in vivo* exposure techniques help the client reduce these excessive or unnecessary behaviors and collect this missing information.

Together, response prevention and *in vivo* exposure weaken associations between behavioral coping responses and anxiety's physiological mobilization. Response prevention (Foa & Kozak, 1986) is used to eliminate excessive fight behaviors; it involves the client's tolerating the anxiety that comes from inaction or overreaction in the face of fear. *In vivo* exposure is used to confront flight and freeze behaviors; it involves the client's tolerating the anxiety of approaching or acting in the face of danger. To maximize client compliance with *in vivo* exposure, a graded approach is used. That is, the client is taught to break down emotionally overwhelming situations into smaller, less anxiety-provoking items. Those items are then ranked from least to most anxiety-provoking. *In vivo* exposure is then carried out, starting with the least anxiety-provoking item. Exposure to that item is repeated until all unnecessary physiological mobilization subsides before the client and therapist move on to the next item. In this way, hypotheses regarding feared outcomes are directly tested. Response prevention follows a similar graded approach, except that the items arranged in a hierarchy are nonadaptive coping behaviors that the client is trying *not* to perform. Both techniques build the client's sense of mastery and confidence in abilities to cope.

Only through repeated experiences that feared consequences do not occur without the execution of coping behaviors will the client be able to acknowledge fully that these behaviors are superfluous. This exposure process erodes the behavioral maintenance of high levels of arousal associated with worry. Table 7.1 summarizes the behaviors to be targeted with the specific techniques recommended. The balance of this chapter details how to implement the three techniques of response prevention, *in vivo* exposure, and pleasurable activity scheduling.

RESPONSE PREVENTION

As listed in Table 7.2, response prevention with clients involves the following 10 steps:

Step 1: Identifying Problem Coping Behaviors

Excessive coping behaviors can be more subtle and difficult to detect in clients with GAD than in those with other anxiety disorders. But problem behaviors can be differentiated from adaptive behaviors by their functional significance. A first step is to review the client's Worry Episode Logs (both the assessment and treatment versions), but it may or may not be apparent from these logs which behaviors are nonadaptive or excessive. A cost–benefit analysis of coping responses (see Chapter 5) can be carried out to assist in this determination. Coping behaviors where costs outweigh benefits are to be targeted in this exercise.

TABLE 7.1. Typical Behavioral Responses and Recommended Treatments in GAD

Behavioral responses	Recommended treatments

Flight and freeze behaviors
  Avoidance
  Procrastination
  Evasion
  Escape
  Inhibition
	In vivo exposure

Fight behaviors
  Over preparation
  Excessive checking
  Overprotection
	Response prevention

Other problematic behaviors
  Reassurance seeking (excessive or unnecessary
  requests for support, assistance or advice)
	Response prevention and/or *in vivo* exposure

Lack of pleasurable activities	Pleasurable activity scheduling

TABLE 7.2. Steps in Implementing Response Prevention

Developing the hierarchy of GAD behaviors

1. Identify problem coping behaviors (from Worry Episode Logs, cost–benefit analysis).
2. Present technique's rationale to client (using cost–benefit analysis).
3. Have client estimate anxiety level (on 0–8 scale) when refraining from coping behaviors in various situations.
4. Sequence anxiety-rated situations into a hierarchy from least to most anxiety-provoking.

Preparing the client for the exercise

5. Select the first response prevention exercise by choosing a less anxiety-provoking situation (e.g., anxiety ranking of 2 or 3).
6. Client identifies automatic images, thoughts, assumptions, and/or beliefs that arise (or are likely to arise) when coping behaviors are withheld in the selected situation.
7. Client generates alternative hypotheses and rational responses.
8. Prepare client to expect:
   a. Initial increase in anxiety.
   b. Plateau.
   c. Dropoff of anxiety to at least half the highest level.

Discussing, assigning, reviewing, and repeating the exercise

9. Discuss where, when, and how to practice on a specific hierarchy item. Then assign this practice as homework to be carried out and recorded at least three times a week between sessions.
10. Review outcomes of the exercise. Have client repeat exercise for the same item until the highest level of anxiety experienced during the exercise is 0 or 1; only then should client move on to the next most anxiety-provoking item in the hierarchy.

Step 2: Present the Rationale for the Technique to the Client

Once the high costs of problem behaviors are established, response prevention can be introduced to the client in terms of its costs and benefits. The therapist can acknowledge that coping behaviors are effective in briefly reducing anxiety. But they are not truly necessary, since anxiety dissipates naturally when problem coping behaviors are withheld. However, to achieve significant reductions in the anxiety over the long term, anxiety evoked by worry stimuli must be tolerated until it has substantially dissipated.

Steps 3 and 4: Putting Problem Coping Behaviors into a Hierarchy

The client estimates his or her anxiety level when refraining from the coping behaviors in various conditions. Then these behaviors are arranged in a graded hierarchy according to these estimates. If the client can only identify high-anxiety situations, the probability of successful completion is low. The therapist should attempt to break these very distressing situations down into smaller steps that are less anxiety-provoking. Or there may be variations on a situation that lessen the anxiety it arouses. The goal is to arrive at a list with items in the 2, 3, or 4 range (on the usual 0–8 scale), as well as higher-level items.

Step 5: Selecting a Low-Level Item from the Hierarchy for Assignment

Once the hierarchy is complete, the therapist and client can select an item from it for the response prevention exercise. Items with low anxiety levels should be selected first, to maximize the probability of success. The therapist and client must be careful to select items where the client's desire to approach is greater than or equal to the desire to avoid the exercise. Items with anxiety ratings of 2 or 3 are ideal, but the first item should be rated no higher than 4.

Steps 6 and 7: Preparing for Problematic Cognition

Worry can be evoked as the client is prepared for the exercise. When this occurs, the therapist can use it as an example of what is likely to occur before and/or during the planned exercise, and can treat it as an opportunity to practice cognitive techniques. The client can be asked to identify the images, thoughts, assumptions, and/or beliefs that arise (or may arise); to generate plausible alternative viewpoints; and to develop rational responses to any problematic cognitions. The client can be asked to use decatastrophization to counter any cognitive avoidance. A cost–benefit analysis can be done if there are doubts about client motivation.

Step 8: Preparing for the Experience of Anxiety during the Assignment

The therapist tells the client what to expect. When the specific coping behaviors are withheld, the initial experience is increased anxiety. After this increase, the anxiety plateaus. After a period of time, ranging from 15 minutes to an hour or two, the anxiety begins to drop. This drop in anxiety occurs naturally, as the parasympathetic nervous system counteracts the sympathetic nervous system. When the level of anxiety has dropped to at least 50% of the highest rate, the exercise is considered complete. At this lower level, the client can much more easily continue to resist acting. But if the client stops the exercise by resuming problematic coping behaviors (particularly when anxiety levels are still high), it will result in a missed treatment opportunity. If the exercise is stopped when anxiety levels are still high, the same (or possibly a higher) anxiety level will be experienced when the exercise is repeated in the future.

Step 9: Discussing and Assigning the Exercise

The therapist and client should discuss the specifics of when, where, and how the item is to be practiced between sessions in the following week. The client should complete the exercise at least three times over the following week and record specifics of the exercise on Handout 7.1. If possible, the first exercise can be done within the session.

Step 10: Reviewing and Repeating the Exercise before Selecting New Items on the Hierarchy

At the next session (and subsequent sessions as necessary), the therapist and client review the outcomes of the exercise. The response prevention exercise is repeated until the highest level of anxiety experienced during the exercise is consistently rated as 0 or 1. Only after this occurs should the client move to the next item on the hierarchy. When clients complete exercises, they are actively working on lowering their overall level of anxiety and building up tolerance of anxiety. The effect of each practice is cumulative. When there is a long delay between response prevention exercises, anxiety levels may increase somewhat. The level can be reduced, however, by simply repeating the exercises closer in time.

The following clinical vignette is an example of setting up a response prevention exercise with a client. (Once again, the client is Richard.)

THERAPIST: One of the behaviors that you have identified as excessive is repeated checking of your work papers for errors. Is that right?

CLIENT: Yes. Although I've been told that my work is superb, I've been criticized for the hours that I bill for my work [cost of checking]. I just take way too long to complete assignments. I have a really hard time giving my work papers to my boss before I consider them perfect in every respect.

THERAPIST: What do you mean when you say, "I have a really hard time"?

CLIENT: I feel so much anxiety about giving them to my boss unless I've gone over them numerous times.

THERAPIST: Have you ever tried to turn your papers in after going through them only once or twice? [Asking about functional significance of checking]

HANDOUT 7.1. Record of Response Prevention Exercise

RECORD OF RESPONSE PREVENTION EXERCISE

Day/date/time: _____

					Anxiety scale			
0	1	2	3	4	5	6	7	8
None		Mild		Moderate		Severe		Extreme

Describe behaviors resisted and situation: _____

_____

Anxiety level at starting time: ____

Maximum anxiety level during exercise: ____

Anxiety level at ending time: ____

Total time spent on exercise: _____

Comments: _____

_____

CLIENT: Never. I would feel incredibly anxious that something was wrong. That would be intolerable.

THERAPIST: How long do you think your anxiety would last?

CLIENT: (*Pause*) . . . I have no idea. It probably would keep getting worse and worse. I don't think I could take it.

THERAPIST: It sounds like you believe that the anxiety would be unending or might spiral out of control. Is that right?

CLIENT: Yes. I guess that's right.

THERAPIST: What do you feel after you check your work?

CLIENT: I feel better.

THERAPIST: Does that feeling last?

CLIENT: For a while, but I usually get anxious when I think about giving my work to my boss. The anxiety only goes away if I've checked it repeatedly and not found any errors.

THERAPIST: It sounds like you believe that the only way you can control your anxiety and worry in this situation is to repeatedly check your work. Is that right?

CLIENT: Yes. That's right.

THERAPIST: Today I'm going to introduce you to a technique called "response prevention." Response prevention exercises allow you to gather concrete evidence to answer the question of whether or not it is in your best interest to continue so much checking.

You have noticed that when certain triggers—like your work papers—spur worry, responses such as excessive checking can be used to neutralize the worry [benefit of checking]. Although you feel soothed after checking your work papers, you've noticed that the anxiety returns after a while [limit of benefit]. You also mentioned that you believe your anxiety will spiral upward if you don't check and can only be controlled by checking [benefit of checking].

CLIENT: That's right.

THERAPIST: I want to remind you of something that we discussed earlier. One fact is that anxiety does not spiral out of control [disputing benefit of checking]. Remember that our bodies have a built-in protection with the sympathetic and parasympathetic nervous systems. After experiencing anxiety for a prolonged period, our bodies naturally enter a restful state. If you were to refrain from checking your papers, eventually you would find that your body relaxed on its own. In other words, too much checking takes up your time and causes problems with your boss. What if you don't really need to do it to keep anxiety under control?

The benefit of doing response prevention is that the exercises allow you to have a firsthand experience of the fact that your body eventually relaxes even when you do not engage in these behaviors. The technique involves taking some small risks by preventing yourself from checking. I want you to be aware that the exercises require you to tolerate some anxiety [disadvantages of response prevention]. To gain benefit from the exercises, the anxiety must be tolerated until the level of anxiety drops to at least half of the highest level. But we can regulate how much anxiety you'll experience during an exercise by picking a behavior according to the amount of anxiety you would experience while resisting the urge to repeatedly check. Does this technique sound like something that you might be willing to try?

CLIENT: (*Pause*) . . . I guess so. Sure.

THERAPIST: Good. Let's talk some more about your work papers. Does excessive checking apply to all sorts of documents?

CLIENT: Yes . . . everything. Memos, letters, briefs . . .

THERAPIST: Would there be any difference in your level of anxiety, depending upon the type of document, if you were to turn in that document in a less perfect form?

CLIENT: Yes. Memos would be the easiest, then letters, then briefs.

THERAPIST: How many memos do you turn in each week?

CLIENT: About three.

THERAPIST: OK. Let's talk some more about the memos. What would you consider a necessary and reasonable number of times to check a memo?

CLIENT: Once the legal research is completed and I've written a first draft, one edit should be sufficient.

THERAPIST: OK. How much anxiety do you think you would experience, on a 0–8 scale, if you resisted the urge to continue checking and turned it in to your boss at that point?

CLIENT: Probably a 3.

THERAPIST: What types of thoughts or images likely are to occur under these circumstances? [Identifying problematic cognitions when coping behaviors are withheld, and generating alternatives]

CLIENT: I probably would be worrying that I made a serious error and have an image of losing my job as a result. But, realistically, I know that losing my job as the result of an error in an internal memo is unlikely.

THERAPIST: What are the realistic odds of this happening?

CLIENT: I guess 0, practically speaking.

THERAPIST: What do you think would be the most likely result?

CLIENT: I probably would be somewhat embarrassed if my boss pointed out an error.

THERAPIST: How long do you think that embarrassment might last?

CLIENT: Maybe half a day if it was a really stupid error.

THERAPIST: Do you think that the cost of that possible embarrassment would be worth the benefit of getting your work out more quickly? [Conducting a cost–benefit analysis]

CLIENT: Yes, definitely. There's no question that the benefits would be greater. My boss would be happier if I were more productive. My wife and kids would be happier with me, too, because I would have more free time.

THERAPIST: So you're saying that if you were to resist checking your memos more than once before turning them in to your boss over the next week, you probably would have to sit through some increased anxiety at first, due to thoughts that you may have made serious errors that will cost you your job. Sitting through this anxiety and eventually getting feedback from your boss would allow you to experience the outcome of not engaging in the extra checking behaviors. You said that the most realistic outcome is that nothing catastrophic will happen, like losing your job. The worst actual outcome would be that you would have to tolerate some anxiety and embarrassment if you made a big error. The most likely positive outcome is that you will be able to get your work papers out more quickly. Is that right? [Preparing the client for what to expect]

CLIENT: Yes. That's right.

THERAPIST: Do you think that you could refrain from more than one edit before turning in your memos to your boss over the next week? This means that you could not retrieve the memo to recheck at any point after the first edit. You would have to be willing to sit through the anxiety until it eventually subsides and wait for feedback from your boss. [Discussing when, where, and how to practice response prevention on a particular item]

CLIENT: Yes, I think I could do that.

THERAPIST: OK. Let's start with memos for your first response prevention exercises. Your assignment, then, is to turn in all of your memos after only one check over the next week. [Assigning the exercise as homework]

CLIENT: OK.

THERAPIST: As you repeat this exercise over and over and experience the positive outcomes, you will notice your anxiety lessening. Eventually, this stimulus will no longer propel these behaviors. It is important to remind yourself that every time you have the urge to recheck your work, and you do not act on this urge and tolerate the anxiety instead, you increase your ability to control your anxiety. Ultimately, these exercises will free you from behaviors that are interfering with your potential to live a happier and more productive life.

At the next session, Richard reported that he was able to complete the assignment successfully. His levels of anxiety were as he expected: The levels of anxiety were most intense right after he turned in the memos to his boss, but he noticed that the anxiety subsided within an hour on each occasion. Richard was able to leave work an hour early three nights that week, although he noticed some worry related to the assignment while at home on those evenings. He used the CR exercises to counter these episodes of worry. Richard observed from his boss's comments that he had written a couple of awkward sentences and had only typographical errors otherwise. By the end of the week, his boss praised him on his quick turn-around time, and his wife expressed happiness that he was spending more time at home.

IN VIVO EXPOSURE

As listed in Table 7.3, *in vivo* exposure with clients involves the following seven steps:

Step 1: Identifying Problematic Flight and Freeze Behaviors Associated with Specific Stimuli

The therapist and client must identify specific flight and freeze behaviors (e.g., avoidance, procrastination, evasion, escape, indecision, or inhibition of activity) that are maintaining excessive worry. This can be done through direct inquiry about these behaviors and by examining the client's Worry Episode Logs for these behaviors. The stimulus events that trigger these behaviors also need to be identified.

Step 2: Identifying More Adaptive Responses to Those Stimuli

After flight/freeze behaviors and stimulus events are identified, the client must identify more adaptive behaviors for coping with those specific stimulus events. These behaviors will tend to involve approaching rather than avoiding the trigger situations, and acting rather than suspending action. As in response prevention, a cost–benefit analysis of coping responses can be used to differentiate adaptive from nonadaptive behaviors and to motivate clients for facing and tolerating their anxiety.

Step 3: Estimating Anxiety Levels Associated with Adaptive Behaviors, and Sequencing Behaviors Hierarchically

After adaptive behaviors are identified, the client must rate the level of anxiety (on the usual 0–8 scale) associated with the execution of specific adaptive behaviors in response to specific stimulus events. If anxiety levels are all rated as high, the behavioral approach toward certain events

---

TABLE 7.3. Steps in Implementing *In Vivo* Exposure

1. Identify problematic flight and freeze behaviors associated with specific stimuli.
2. Identify more adaptive behaviors to those stimuli (using cost–benefit analysis).
3. Estimate anxiety levels associated with adaptive behaviors, and sequence behaviors hierarchically.
4. Select item for *in vivo* exposure.
5. Predict outcomes of exposure to identify and prepare for problematic cognitions.
6. Assign exposure.
7. Review exercise and have client repeat as necessary before selecting new exposure assignments.

---

should be broken down into smaller, less anxiety-provoking behavioral steps. These behavioral steps are arranged in a hierarchy.

Step 4: Selecting an Item for *In Vivo* Exposure

Once the hierarchy is complete, the therapist and client select an item with a low anxiety level for *in vivo* exposure. The item's anxiety level should be no higher than 4. At higher levels, the desire to avoid is greater than the desire to approach. Lower levels of anxiety increase the probability that the client will execute approach behavior.

Step 5: Predicting Outcomes of Exposure

Prior to the exposure, the therapist should have the client make specific predictions concerning the outcomes of the exposure. Through this process, automatic images, thoughts, assumptions, and beliefs associated with confronting the event can be identified and queried, and alternative viewpoints and rational responses can be generated.

Step 6: Assigning Exposure

The client is given the assignment to engage in this behavior prior to the next session. If the approach behavior can be executed repeatedly, at least three exposures should be done between sessions.

Step 7: Reviewing and Repeating the Exercise before Selecting New Exposure Assignments

The therapist and client review the results of the exposures with respect to the predictions. Cost–benefit analysis of specific coping responses may also be reviewed. Approach behaviors are repeated until the highest level of anxiety during those exposures is rated 0 or 1. Only then should the client move on to items in the hierarchy associated with higher levels of anxiety.

Confronting frequently avoided situations raises anxiety levels at first. Again, the therapist will need to assure the client that this increase is temporary when flight and freeze behaviors cannot be rationally or reasonably supported. When the client follows through with approach behaviors despite the anxiety, a significant drop in the level of anxiety is eventually noticed.

An example of setting up an *in vivo* exposure with Richard is provided below.

THERAPIST: You mentioned that you've been procrastinating over speaking with your boss about taking a vacation. What level of anxiety, on a 0–8 scale, would you experience if you were to walk into your boss's office to make that request right now?

CLIENT: Probably 6 [too high for initial exposure].

THERAPIST: What do you do to procrastinate? [Identifying problematic flight behaviors]

CLIENT: When my wife mentions a vacation, I find myself walking out of the room, trying to change the subject, or making excuses as to why it can't be done in the near future. . . . I feel like doing the same here.

THERAPIST: What would be the advantage of avoiding this topic right now? [Conducting a cost–benefit analysis]

CLIENT: I would feel less anxious.

THERAPIST: Permanently?

CLIENT: No. Just right now.

THERAPIST: Are there any other advantages?

CLIENT: If I don't go on vacation, I don't have to worry about someone covering my assignments and outperforming me. [Predicting a problematic outcome]

THERAPIST: Is that worry realistic?

CLIENT: (*Pause*) . . . I guess not. I'm one of the top performers, but that's partly because I work so hard.

THERAPIST: Are there any other advantages?

CLIENT: I can't think of any others.

THERAPIST: What are the disadvantages of avoiding a vacation?

CLIENT: Well, my wife is getting pretty upset with me. I'm not spending enough time with her or the kids.

THERAPIST: Are there any other disadvantages?

CLIENT: I need a break. I'm worried that I'll burn myself out if I don't take a break.

THERAPIST: And then what?

CLIENT: I could run myself into a state of exhaustion and eventually get fired or sick. I know I can't keep up this relentless pace without any break.

THERAPIST: Right. Taking breaks will maximize your ability to focus on your work and stay positive over longer periods of time. What are some things that you could do to make it possible to take a vacation? [Identifying more adaptive behaviors]

CLIENT: I could sit down with my wife to formulate a vacation plan.

THERAPIST: How much anxiety would you have if you were to do that step only?

CLIENT: I guess about 4 [at the high end for an initial exposure].

THERAPIST: Are there other steps that would be less anxiety-provoking?

CLIENT: I could look at my calendar and decide the best dates for going away.

THERAPIST: How much anxiety would you experience if you carried out this step only?

CLIENT: Between 2 and 3.

THERAPIST: What are the advantages of taking these behavioral steps, instead of avoiding?

CLIENT: I would finally take a vacation. My wife and kids would be happy. I would feel better. I would feel more refreshed and energized in relation to my work. I wouldn't have to worry about this any more.

THERAPIST: What are the disadvantages of taking these behavioral steps?

CLIENT: I would feel some anxiety . . . temporarily.

THERAPIST: Do you want to begin taking steps toward this goal of taking a vacation, one step at a time? We could start right now with you looking at your calendar.

CLIENT: OK . . . but I'm feeling anxious.

THERAPIST: Rate your anxiety.

CLIENT: It's a 3.

THERAPIST: Try to stick with what we're doing, despite this feeling. The feelings of anxiety eventually will dissipate if you persist.

CLIENT: Are you sure?

THERAPIST: Yes. If you stick with this, the anxiety eventually will dissipate.

CLIENT: OK.

THERAPIST: What do you need to do to make a decision about the dates for a vacation?

CLIENT: Check my calendar for important dates related to various work assignments.

THERAPIST: Can you do this now? [Assigning the exposure]

CLIENT: Yes . . . (takes out calendar and begins to check dates).

THERAPIST: And?

CLIENT: (Pause) . . . I don't know . . . I'm not sure . . . It doesn't look like any time is a good time.

THERAPIST: Stick with it. Keep looking. . . .

CLIENT: I really don't see any time that's good. This new guy in the office is really a whiz. If he takes over my assignments, my boss may decide to replace me. [problematic cognitions]

THERAPIST: What is your goal right now?

CLIENT: Oh, right . . . to look at dates for this vacation.

THERAPIST: Right. You're getting sidetracked from the main issue with a potential problem that you already said was unlikely. Try to let go of that worry and refocus on your goal.

CLIENT: (Pause) . . . I don't know. . . .

THERAPIST: Keep looking. . . .

CLIENT: Maybe the first 2 weeks in April?

THERAPIST: Keep going. . . .

CLIENT: (Pause) . . . OK. Those are the best weeks, the first 2 weeks in April.

THERAPIST: Good. You just accomplished your first goal. How do you feel? [Reviewing the outcomes]

CLIENT: Some relief. I feel better that I finally decided on the dates.

THERAPIST: What is your level of anxiety right now?

CLIENT: I guess about a 1 . . . but now I have to talk to my wife.

THERAPIST: How do you feel about trying the next step of formulating a concrete vacation plan with your wife as the exposure assignment over the next week? [Assigning new exposure]

CLIENT: That's making it a lot closer to reality.

THERAPIST: We are not speaking about the last step of talking to your boss. The assignment would be to speak only with your wife about the vacation. The purpose of this exercise would be to sit through the anxiety that is elicited with this step, only.

CLIENT: OK. I can do that.

THERAPIST: Good. I want to warn you that you are going to have similar urges to avoid, just like you did when you took out your calendar. Remember that your anxiety and the urge to avoid will be strong in the beginning. Also, remember that if you sit through this anxiety with the urge to avoid, and purposefully focus back on your main goal, the anxiety eventually will dissipate. Stick with the assignment until you notice that your anxiety is half the amount that it was at the beginning.

PLEASURABLE ACTIVITY SCHEDULING

As noted earlier, individuals with GAD often exhibit reduced participation in pleasurable activities. This may be due to the facts that excessive worry and coping diminish the time and attention available to these activities, and/or that underlying negative beliefs exist about these activities (e.g., "I won't be in control of my work responsibilities if I take off time to have fun with my family"). Deficits in planning, scheduling, and executing activities that are pleasurable can exacerbate the difficulties with controlling worry, because there is no alternative focus for attention and action. The technique of scheduling pleasurable activities counteracts these deficits and provides adaptive alternatives. This technique was originally developed by Lewinsohn (1975).

Identifying pleasurable activities

Some clients may already be aware of activities that they find pleasurable, but others may need assistance with identifying these activities. The Pleasurable Activity Log (see Handout 7.2; Figure 3.3 in Chapter 3 is a filled-in version of this handout) may be useful for identifying these activities. With clients who are relatively unaware of what they find pleasurable, the therapist can explore activities that the clients may have enjoyed during other periods of their lives (e.g., childhood, adolescence, or college). The therapist can explore aspects of current activities (e.g., taking care of kids, business engagements) for elements of pleasure (e.g., playing ball, chatting about current events). Alternative activities can be identified that also contain these elements of pleasure without the obligations or responsibilities of the current activities. If a client is at a complete loss, the therapist can present a wide array of options to the client and ask what sounds appealing. The client may need to sample a variety of activities and observe whether or not he or she experiences pleasure and desires to repeat the activity.

PLEASURABLE ACTIVITY LOG

Intensity of pleasure

0	1	2	3	4	5	6	7	8
None		Low		Moderate		High		Extreme

Date	Activity	Duration	Rating	Comments

Implementing the Technique

During initial practices, it is not unusual for clients to experience anxiety while engaging in "pleasurable" activities. When this occurs, ratings of pleasure may be very low, even with activities that have been enjoyed in the past. It is important to forewarn the client of this possible experience during initial practices. As in response prevention and *in vivo* exposure exercises, the anxiety dissipates with repeated practice. Ratings of pleasure typically increase as anxiety subsides. It is important that the client tolerate the anxiety until this occurs. If the client is testing an activity for pleasure, the client should refrain from evaluating the activity until anxiety levels are extremely low or nonexistent. If the experience of the activity at that point is evaluated as negative or neutral, the client should eliminate this activity and experiment with a new activity.

Pleasurable activity scheduling involves the following steps:

1. Identify potentially pleasurable activities.
2. Have the client choose one of these activities for experimentation.
3. Determine whether engaging in this activity requires preliminary steps. If so, identify those steps.
4. Set up a concrete schedule for carrying out the activity (including preliminary steps, if required), and give an assignment to be completed and recorded on the Pleasurable Activity Log (Handout 7.2) by the following session.
5. Identify cognitions (thoughts, images, assumptions, beliefs) associated with the execution of that activity. (Utilize CR exercises where appropriate.)
6. Review the results of the assignment in the next session.

The following clinical vignette gives an example of implementation of this technique with Richard. (Richard is about to go on his April vacation.)

THERAPIST: What kinds of things will you do on vacation?

CLIENT: My wife usually makes the plans. I'm not sure.

THERAPIST: What would you like to do?

CLIENT: Well, we're going to stay in a resort. There should be a lot of nice things to do.

THERAPIST: Like what?

CLIENT: Golf. Tennis. Swimming. Horseback riding. Boating.

THERAPIST: Do you plan on doing any of these activities?

CLIENT: I don't know. . . . I usually take my computer so I can work on my investments. I call in to work a couple times a day. Sometimes they need my help on certain projects, so I do it on my computer in the hotel room.

THERAPIST: It sounds like you're planning to continue going to work, but in your hotel room instead of your office.

CLIENT: I guess so.

THERAPIST: What does your wife do?

CLIENT: She plays with the kids. It's a break for her not to cook and clean. It's a lot easier with all the fun activities for the kids.

THERAPIST: But what about you? Don't you need a break?

CLIENT: Yes.

THERAPIST: So . . . what kinds of pleasurable activities will you do, either alone or with your wife or with your family?

CLIENT: I haven't really thought about it.

THERAPIST: What do you like to do?

CLIENT: I like to golf, swim, play tennis, boat . . . that's partly why we picked this resort.

THERAPIST: How about thinking of organizing your time to make sure you do these things? What would you need to do?

CLIENT: I would have to put away my computer and not call in to work. But what if there's a problem at work? I feel anxious about not being in touch.

THERAPIST: What kind of problem could arise at work?

CLIENT: There could be an emergency that requires my involvement.

THERAPIST: How could you structure things so that you prioritize your vacation over your work, but make it possible for the office to get in touch with you if absolutely necessary?

CLIENT: I could put the responsibility to call on them. I could tell them to call only if it's an emergency that absolutely no one else can handle.

THERAPIST: Good. How could you structure your time for pleasurable activity?

CLIENT: I could plan to golf in the morning and swim or boat with my kids in the afternoon.

THERAPIST: Does the resort have structured activities for kids that could give you free time to spend with your wife?

CLIENT: Yeah, they do . . . my wife and I could play tennis, maybe go out to lunch or dinner alone. This is sounding good.

THERAPIST: How about setting up a concrete plan to make sure this happens?

CLIENT: OK.

THERAPIST: Do you have a calendar with you that includes the dates of your vacation?

CLIENT: Yes.

THERAPIST: I want you to take out this calendar right now and make a schedule for your pleasurable activities. You are to put down pleasurable activities for good weather and backup activities for bad weather. Schedule one pleasurable activity for the morning, one for the afternoon, and one for the evening. For example, you might schedule a tennis game with your wife in the morning, swimming with your family in the afternoon, and playing miniature golf with the family in the evening. The backup plan might be to take the family shopping in the resort's town in the morning, go bowling in the afternoon, and go to a movie in the evening. An activity does not have to require a lot of energy. It can be very quiet and relaxed, such as simply sitting in a beach chair and watching, listening, feeling, and smelling the ocean and the ocean breeze.

CLIENT: OK. . . . (*Richard takes out the calendar and fills it out for every day of his vacation.*)

THERAPIST: May I look at what you wrote?

CLIENT: Sure (*shows calendar to therapist*).

THERAPIST: I'm going to make a copy of this calendar at the end of our session. You may want to modify the schedule of activities with your wife and kids. How do you think you'll feel doing these activities?

CLIENT: I'll probably feel anxious when I do these things. Taking time to have fun is so unlike me.

THERAPIST: You are very likely to experience anxiety at first. If you stick with each activity and wait for the anxiety to pass, you eventually will begin to enjoy yourself. You have to persist with the activity, despite the anxiety, for this to occur.

CLIENT: I'm glad we made a plan for my communication with the office. Knowing that my boss and colleagues will be responsible for staying on top of things while I'm away releases me from a big burden.

THERAPIST: Can you think of anything else that might worry you?

CLIENT: (*Pause*) . . . Not at the moment, but I'm sure something will come up.

THERAPIST: If anything comes up, you can record it in the "Comments" section of the Pleasurable Activity Log. I want you to record your participation in each of your selected activities on this log at the end of every day throughout your vacation. Bring the log sheets to our next session.

CLIENT: OK.

At the next session, Richard reported this vacation as one of his best and most relaxing. His logs indicated little pleasure on the first day of vacation (pleasure ratings were about 2 on every activity). His comments indicated that he had to tolerate moderate to severe anxiety at the beginning of each of these activities on this first day. Over the course of the week, however, his pleasure ratings climbed and were consistently high by the last 2 days. Fortunately, there were no work emergencies to interrupt the vacation.

CHAPTER EIGHT

Supplementary Treatment Techniques

The techniques presented in this chapter are intended to enhance treatment outcome for those who are not showing an adequate response to the research-based cognitive-behavioral therapy (CBT) techniques presented earlier. These additional techniques for GAD are still being tested in the context of new treatment packages. The rationales for their inclusion in such packages are based on (1) basic research on worry, (2) studies of worry in GAD, and/or (3) research on characteristics of clients who do not respond to standard CBT. Although outcome research is still in progress, we decided to include a chapter on these techniques, on the basis of our clinical impressions that many of these techniques are likely to improve treatment outcomes. Because a strong base of treatment outcome research is not yet available, we recommend that these techniques be reserved for those who are at high risk of a poor treatment response (e.g., notable interpersonal problems), or who exhibit a poor treatment response to or recurrent relapses with standard CBT. We present the techniques under the rubrics of mindfulness, emotional processing and regulation training, interpersonal effectiveness, and time management (see Table 8.1).

TABLE 8.1. Techniques That Target Associated Problems

Problems	Techniques
Experiential avoidance	Mindfulness
Emotion regulation	Emotional processing and regulation training
Interpersonal problems	Interpersonal effectiveness
Mismanagement of time	Time management

MINDFULNESS

In recent years, mindfulness has been applied with a wide variety of disorders, such as borderline personality disorder (Linehan, 1993a), substance abuse (Hayes, Strosahl, & Wilson, 1999), trauma (Follette, 1994), and depression (Teasdale et al., 2000). Roemer and Orsillo (2002) have introduced mindfulness as a potentially effective component in the treatment of GAD. Roemer and Orsillo argue that GAD is characterized by "experiential avoidance," which is both strategic and automatic avoidance of internal distress. This conceptualization of GAD stems from Borkovec's notion of, and research on, worry as a form of motivated avoidance of emotional imagery and arousal. Roemer and Orsillo (2002) and Orsillo, Roemer, and Barlow (2003) have proposed a treatment model with acceptance-based techniques of mindfulness drawn from dialectical behavior therapy (Linehan, 1993a, 1993b), and techniques of mindful action drawn from acceptance and commitment therapy for substance abuse (Hayes et al., 1999). Their treatment package also incorporates elements from Borkovec's version of CBT for GAD (Borkovec & Roemer, 1994) and Zinbarg, Craske, and Barlow's (1993) treatment package in *Mastering Your Anxiety and Worry*. Roemer and Orsillo's treatment for GAD directly targets experiential avoidance and the habitual restrictions in action that are associated with GAD. Their specific treatment package consists of four components: (1) psychoeducation; (2) mindfulness, early cue detection, and monitoring; (3) relaxation/ mindfulness techniques; and (4) mindful action (which integrates other behavioral treatment strategies for increasing effective action under difficult conditions). The research on the effectiveness of their treatment for GAD is still in the preliminary stages. In addition, there is notable theoretical debate as to why mindfulness might be effective in the treatment of GAD (Wells, 2002; Craske & Hazlett-Stevens, 2002) and of the other anxiety disorders (Craske & Hazlett-Stevens, 2002). It is with these cautions and concerns in mind that we discuss the use of mindfulness within treatment.

Training in mindfulness presumably strengthens a person's abilities to process immediate experience more fully. As such, it has the potential for enhancing many of the standard CBT techniques for GAD (e.g., scheduled worry time, hypothesis testing, worry exposure, etc.). In addition, it has the potential for enhancing Wells's (1995) treatment package for GAD, which specifically requires clients to "let go" of worry in order to challenge metaworry, and Ladouceur, Blais, Freeston, and Dugas's (1998) package, which requires cognitive exposure to threatening images while using covert response prevention (see Chapter 1). Mindfulness is also part of Newman, Castonguay, Borkovec, and Molnar's (2004) newly developed treatment package for clients with GAD and interpersonal difficulties (discussed later in this chapter). In this section, we present a general discussion of mindfulness and how to develop mindfulness skills. For more detailed information on how to teach and learn mindfulness, including further client handouts, we refer readers to Linehan (1993b) and Segal, Williams, and Teasdale (2002).

Mindfulness is a form of meditation from Eastern spiritual traditions. It requires the development of three key qualities in one's attention: (1) withholding of judgment, (2) intentional awareness, and (3) a focus on the present moment. Focusing attention on the present moment allows the individual to fully process all aspects of immediate experience, which include all cognitive, physiological, and/or behavioral activities. Mindfulness can be thought of as an internal, on-the-spot self-monitoring tool. Like other self-monitoring tools, it helps make automatic processing more conscious. When applied to emotional experience, mindfulness can be used simply to allow this experience to occur, thus interrupting avoidance responses to internally generated perceived threats. This may be particularly useful when the perceived threats are related to natural mental and physical processes, such as worry and arousal. Rather than recording automatic processes on a log or diary, the client is trained to purposefully observe, accept, and verbally label his or her moment-by-moment experience. Through this process, the client can become aware of faulty associations between this experience and threat. The therapist can explain mindfulness to the client as follows:

"Much of the time, we are not fully aware of our moment-to-moment experience. We go through much of life automatically. We can easily fall into habits of sensing and reacting to experience, with only a small part of our awareness. For example, we can drive our car on a familiar highway without full awareness, and we can miss our intended exit if it's not the usual one. But we can learn to control our attention and become aware of automatic patterns with mindfulness skills. Mindfulness is about noticing your unfiltered experience of reality—of what really is, right now, in the present moment.

"Practicing mindfulness requires you to withhold judgment. We all have a natural tendency to evaluate and judge our experience. We attach meanings to it. But judgment and meaning can get in the way of seeing what is really there. In mindfulness we actively detach these evaluations, meanings, and judgments from experience. All experience is accepted, and all judgments are 'let go.' 'Acceptance' here does not mean that you must approve or like something. It only means acknowledging or admitting the reality of your experience. Reality is filled with obstacles and unpleasant situations. We must first acknowledge that they are there if we are ever to improve things.

" 'Mindfulness' means intentional awareness. You choose to focus your attention on a particular experience and keep your attention there. This is more difficult than it seems and takes practice. The mind has a habit of wandering when we are trying to pay attention. Much of mindfulness practice is about noticing when the mind has wandered, then gently bringing it back to the present moment. Notice where the mind has gone, but don't judge; just bring your attention back to where it was.

"Awareness naturally wanders or veers away from the present moment. When we 'space out' (as with boredom), we leave present experience. When we hold on to experience (as with pleasure), we leave the present moment. When we fight against or run away from experience (as with discomfort), we leave the present. Staying in the moment means continually coming back to the present as a new moment. It does not mean trying to prevent the mind from wandering; rather, it is a process of becoming aware of the wandering of one's mind and then gently bringing the mind back into the moment. Staying present in the moment is a continual series of new beginnings. No matter where the mind may wander at any point in time, the process is one of continually bringing one's mind into the present."

A version of this introduction to mindfulness can be given to the client as Handout 8.1. Segal et al. (2002) introduce clients in groups to mindfulness practice through what they call

HANDOUT 8.1. About Mindfulness

ABOUT MINDFULNESS

We go through much of life automatically, not fully aware of our experience. We can fall easily into habits of sensing and reacting, and so we stop paying attention. We can drive on the highway without paying attention when it's a routine habit. If we drive the same route with a new destination, though, we can miss our turnoff if we aren't paying attention. Whenever we aren't fully paying attention, we slip into habits from the past and stop noticing what is really there right now. We also can miss many of life's pleasures.

"Mindfulness" simply means paying attention to (1) your direct experience, (2) in the present moment, (3) without judging. When you are mindful, you are aware on purpose and paying attention. There is no goal except awareness of the present moment. Let's look in turn at what the three mindfulness qualities mean.

YOUR DIRECT EXPERIENCE

Direct experience is anything you can directly sense here and now through sight, taste, smell, touch, hearing, or internal physical feeling. We can directly sense thoughts and emotions. But the contents of thoughts and emotions do not necessarily match the present world outside you. When you think about a chair, you experience a thought-chair, not a chair that you can physically sit in at that moment. Thinking about the taste of chocolate is not the same experience as really tasting chocolate. Feeling frightened does not mean that there must really be something to be frightened about. The contents of thoughts and feelings often have to do with the past, with our interpretations of what we directly sense, or with our imagining of the future. These thoughts and feelings may or may not accurately match facts in the real world.

IN THE PRESENT MOMENT

It's hard to keep our awareness in the present. Our attention naturally wanders away from the present moment. When we "space out," we leave the present; we leave direct experience, and we get lost in the contents of our thoughts. The present moment is always changing, and so our experience in the present is always changing. When we try to hold onto a good experience, we leave the present. When we try to fight or flee an uncomfortable sensation, we leave the present. Staying present does not mean trying to stop your mind from wandering. Rather, it means noticing that your mind has wandered and gently bringing it back to the present, over and over again. Staying in the moment means continually coming back to the present as a new moment.

One helpful way to stay in the present is to focus your attention on immediate physical bodily sensations or on your breath. It is also possible to pay attention to the flow of thoughts and feelings in your mind. But this means noticing thoughts as thoughts and feelings as feelings—not getting caught in their contents. It means stepping back and watching thoughts or feelings come and go, followed by others.

(continued)

WITHOUT JUDGING

We have a natural tendency to evaluate and judge our experience. We attach meanings to our experience. We label experiences as "good" or "bad," "right" or "wrong." Mindfulness is a process of observing without evaluating or judging. It is difficult to observe accurately if we immediately judge it in some way. Mindfulness is about paying attention as a basic reality check, and it requires you to suspend all judgments and interpretations. All experience is acknowledged. All judgments are "let go." There is no success or failure. Acknowledging (or "accepting") does not mean approval or liking. It means only that you are aware that this *is* the experience.

MINDFULNESS AND WORRY

Worry is often about trying to solve problems through rational thinking. When this does not work, the mind can go around in circles. Mindfulness is not about solving problems or "doing" anything. It is about stepping out of old patterns. It is about stepping back from the urge to change or fix or think. It is about "being" in the moment—about experiencing the present for its own sake. With practice, mindfulness allows you to notice worry in the moment, but not to get caught in it. It can help you notice the parts of the worry process as they might unfold. You might notice what triggers worry, what thoughts you have when worrying, how your body responds, and what urges arise to act or do something. Mindfulness asks you to notice the urge to act, but it helps you learn that you do not have to act on your urges. Notice the worry thoughts, but do not get caught in the thoughts, or try to shut them out or hold onto them. Allow the worry when it comes; let it go when it goes; notice it, do not judge it.

PRACTICING MINDFULNESS

Practice mindfulness every day of every week for at least 5–20 minutes. You may not learn mindfulness skills well if you practice less than once every day. At the beginning, start to practice mindfulness when your worry levels are low and you are in a place that does not trigger your anxieties. As you become more skillful, practice mindfulness under more difficult conditions.

SOME MINDFULNESS EXERCISES

- Sit for 5 minutes (or longer) with eyes closed, giving your full attention to what you hear. When your attention wanders, notice that, then gently bring it back to what you hear. Continue doing that.
- Slowly eat an apple, paying attention to how it looks; how it feels in your hand and your mouth; how it smells, sounds, and tastes. Keep your attention focused on the experience of the apple from moment to moment as you eat it. When your attention wanders, notice what it is that took your mind away, and then gently bring your mind back to the apple.
- Pick any routine task that you can do without much thinking, and do it while fully paying attention, moment by moment. When your attention wanders, notice where it went, then gently bring your mind back to what you were doing.

"The Raisin Exercise." This is based on an exercise developed by Kabat-Zinn (1990). Everyone in the group is given a raisin to hold in his or her hand. Then the group leader guides participants in slowly and carefully noticing the raisin from a variety of sensory angles: sight (color, shape, texture); smell; touch (texture, weight); and finally the mouth's sensations in tasting, chewing, and swallowing the raisin. A transcript for a similar exercise, based on Segal et al.'s (2002) but using a pretzel, can be found in Table 8.2. Another very useful and simple mindfulness exercise uses the experience of breathing as an anchor for staying aware and in the present. Kabat-Zinn (1990), Linehan (1993b), and Segal et al. (2002) each use mindfulness of breath in this way. Breathing connects us all with fundamental existence. Awareness of one's own breath is a way to bring oneself back into the present moment when awareness has veered

---

TABLE 8.2. The Pretzel Exercise

Instructions:

Place one small pretzel in the client's hand, and then guide the client's attention to as many sensory details as possible, starting with the way the pretzel looks and feels in the hand. Try not to use the word "pretzel." Do not tell the client what you see or what he or she is to see. Instead, simply direct the client's attention to the details of his or her own sensory experience. The following is a suggested transcript.

- Hold out your hand. I am placing something in it. (*Place pretzel in the palm of client's hand.*) Feel it in your palm. (*Pause*)
- Now look at it as if you have never seen anything like it before. Look at it as if you were a child seeing one for the first time. (*Pause*)
- Notice the color. Notice where it is light or dark. Notice how the light strikes it. (*Pause*)
- Using the fingers of your other hand, turn it over. How does this side look? Is it the same as or different from the other side? (*Pause*)
- Using the fingers of your other hand, exploring the surface with your fingertips. Focus on the texture, the smooth or rough. (*Pause*)
- Notice the thoughts that come into your mind while you are doing this. You might think, "This is weird," or "Why are we doing this?" Don't judge the thoughts; anything you think is OK. Just notice them as thoughts. Then bring your awareness back to what is in your hand. (*Pause*)
- Now bring it up under your nose . . . notice the smell each time you breathe in. (*Pause*)
- Bring it to your lips. (*Pause*) Gently lick the surface with your tongue. (*Pause*) Notice the sensations on your tongue as it licks. (*Pause*)
- Gently place it inside your mouth and feel it with your tongue, your mouth. Notice the taste; explore the sensations, textures, and flavors with your tongue. (*Pause*)
- Notice any urge to bite into it, but don't bite until you feel ready. (*Pause*)
- When you bite, . . . notice the tastes released. (*Pause*)
- As you slowly chew, pay attention to the changing texture. (*Pause*)
- Notice when you feel an urge to swallow. Then swallow when you feel ready. (*Pause*)
- Notice the feel of what you've swallowed moving down your throat until the feel begins to fade.

Assignment: Try this practice with different types of food and drink.

Note. Based on Kabat-Zinn (1990) and Segal, Williams, and Teasdale (2002).

away. Mindfulness of breath is particularly useful when one finds oneself in the process of avoiding or fighting against present experience; focusing on one's breath is a coping strategy for breaking through nonpresent awareness and returning to mindfulness. In short, singularly focusing on breath is a visceral way of reconnecting with being in the moment. Handout 8.2 contains instructions for a breathing exercise based on Segal et al. (2002). The handout can be given to clients after it is introduced in session. Note that the handout assumes that clients already know diaphragmatic breathing (DB).

As Segal et al. (2002) explain, another crucial aspect of mindfulness is teaching clients to distinguish reality and sensory perceptions of reality from thoughts, emotions, or interpretations in the mind. Clients learn that they do not need to react immediately to thoughts, emotions, or physical urges. They can simply observe thoughts as thoughts, without getting caught up in the thought content. Urges to act can be noticed and allowed to pass without being acted upon. Handout 8.3 offers instructions for the kind of exercise that can teach clients these general distinctions. For example, when the exercise is introduced, the client can be told that awareness is a window on the mind. Through this window, the mind's inner processes can be noticed and labeled. Thoughts and emotions, can be observed, labeled as thoughts or emotions and then let go without disrupting ongoing experience. The exercise described in Handout 8.4 is specifically designed for mindfully noticing and labeling fear or worry in the moment and then returning to the breath as a way not to get caught up in the worry. Cognitive distortions, physiological mobilization, behavioral urges and actions, and feelings can be noticed and labeled as such while maintaining continual awareness of the breath and immediate experience.

If the therapist decides to train the client in mindfulness, each mindfulness exercise should be done initially in session and then individually assigned for practice between sessions once or twice a day. The various exercises take between 5 and 20 minutes to complete.

Clients should be told to practice mindfulness every day throughout each week, to ensure that the various skills are adequately developed. Less than one practice of a skill per day may interfere with mastering that skill. The initial exercises should be carried out when anxiety levels and exposures to anxiety-provoking stimuli are at a minimum. Later exercises should include practicing mindfulness under more difficult (high-anxiety) conditions.

Clients sometimes report difficulties with focusing attention in the exercises, and/or discomfort with focusing on internal bodily processes. In both instances, the therapist can describe the difficulties as typical in people with GAD. These difficulties do not represent failure or a problem with mastering mindfulness. The therapist can explain that mindfulness is like stepping back to sit in an out-of-the-way chair within one's mind. From the chair, one can observe events. In the beginning, the client may feel restless with sitting in this chair and perhaps not yet comfortable with that position. It is important to practice acceptance of and patience with this restlessness and discomfort. In time, the mind will settle down and begin to feel more comfortable. The exercises can be broken down into smaller segments if the difficulties are extreme (e.g., focusing on one sensation over a shorter duration or one body part or bodily process at a time, and then incrementally extending the exercise).

MINDFULNESS OF BREATH

Paying attention to your breathing is a mindfulness exercise you can do any time, any place. Awareness of your breathing can help anchor your attention, and thus can help steady and calm you. Stay with the practice as best you can for about 15 minutes, or longer if you wish.

- Find a comfortable sitting position. Loosen clothing around your waist if you need to. Gently close your eyes. Rest a hand on your lower abdomen. Breathe through your nose.
- Breathe into your lower abdomen. Feel your hand rise as you breathe in. Feel your hand fall as you breathe out. When you are breathing in this way, remove your hand.
- Notice the air as moves in through your nose.
- Notice the air as it moves out through your nose.
- Follow the breath into your abdomen. Feel it expand.
- Follow the breath out of the abdomen.
- Do not try to change or control the breath in any way. Accept the breath as it is.
- When your mind wanders, this is not a problem. Simply notice where it has been—for example, "worry thoughts." Gently bring your mind back to your lower abdomen. Focus on the physical sensations as your abdomen rises and falls with each breath.
- Over and over again, focus on the breath. When your mind has wandered, notice where it has been. Gently follow the breath to reconnect with the here-and-now.

Assignment: Try this practice in different positions and quiet places.

Note. Based on Segal, Williams, and Teasdale (2002).

MINDFULNESS OF MENTAL EVENTS

- Practice mindful awareness of your breath (see Handout 8.2) for 5–10 minutes.
- When you are ready, let go of the attention to your breath and focus on events in your mind. There is no need to create events in the mind; just let them occur naturally.
- Observe your mind from a distance, as if you were sitting on a riverbank watching the current. It carries things into view and then carries them away out of view. Do not step into the current. Simply observe it and what it carries.
- Wait with attentiveness for thoughts or images as they arise and pass.
- Simply open your awareness as various thoughts and images surface, become clearer, and submerge again and again. Take a few minutes to bring awareness to thoughts and images.

Assignment: Sit in various locations to practice mindfulness of mental events (e.g., on a bus or train, alone in a room at home or in another solitary location, etc.).

Note. Based on Segal, Williams, and Teasdale (2002).

USING MINDFULNESS TO "LET GO" OF WORRY

When you notice worry or fear:

- **Observe and accept.** Focus awareness on your inner experience. Notice what is. Notice thoughts, images, feelings, urges, and bodily sensations. Cling to nothing. Push nothing away. Briefly describe the experiences—"worry thoughts" or "frightening images" or "fearful feelings."

- **Refocus attention on the breath.** Gently refocus attention on the breath. Be aware of the physical sensations of each in-breath, each out-breath. In the back of your mind, note each breath (e.g., "in-breath . . . out-breath," etc.) or count each breath ("in-one . . . out-one, in-two . . . out-two," etc.").

- **Open and expand attention.** Now open and expand your awareness to your whole body. Notice any discomfort or tension and breathe into those places, then breathe out from those places. Whatever you feel is OK. Just notice and breathe.

Note. Based on Segal, Williams, and Teasdale (2002).

EMOTIONAL PROCESSING AND REGULATION TRAINING

Mennin, Heimberg, Turk, and Fresco (2002) have proposed that individuals with GAD have extreme difficulty understanding their emotional experience. They are deficient in skills for regulating that experience, and thus utilize worry excessively as a cognitive strategy to suppress or control their emotional experience. Clearly, any avoidance of emotion (as suggested by Borkovec, Alcaine, & Behar, 2004) would maintain and/or exacerbate such deficiencies.

Preliminary research in Mennin et al.'s (2002) laboratory has provided some support for their proposal. They found that individuals with GAD exhibited more difficulty identifying, describing, and accepting various emotional experiences and were less able to self-soothe with negative emotional experiences. Techniques that increase awareness, understanding, and regulation of emotional experience would counter such deficits.

Based on their research, Mennin et al. (2002) have argued for the inclusion of emotion regulation skills in treatment packages for GAD. They suggest three treatment components to foster skills in emotion regulation: (1) psychoeducation about emotions, (2) emotion evocation techniques, and (3) emotion regulation skill training. This training also would address any avoidance of emotional experience, in that the first two components evoke and deepen emotional experience.

Unfortunately, we could not find any completed treatment outcome research on the inclusion of these techniques in the treatment of GAD. We have chosen to draw from a variety of sources (Greenberg & Safran, 1987; Linehan, a, 1993b: Newman et al., 2004; Young, Klosko, & Weishaar, 2003) for suggested treatment options to address the emotional regulation deficits in GAD. As such, any of these techniques should be used with this caution in mind. Table 8.3 presents a summary of the steps in emotional processing and regulation training.

Step 1: Psychoeducation about Emotions and Rationale for Training

Clients can be given the following information. The key points are summarized in Handout 8.5.

> "We experience a range of different emotions, including love, joy, anger, sadness, fear and anxiety, shame, and guilt. These and other emotions serve useful purposes for us. They signal us and others that our basic needs, concerns, or goals are being either met or not met. They motivate our behavior. They validate our perceptions and interpretations (although sometimes incorrectly). They provide information to others about us. They motivate others' behavior in relation to us. Actions based on emotions can be constructive, destructive, or (more rarely) neutral.

> "People with GAD tend to quell their emotions with worry. They seem to feel that an intense emotion is a 'problem' that needs to be solved. This is different from others, who feel that emotions indicate whether or not their basic needs, concerns, or goals are supported or frustrated by external circumstances. People with GAD often try to think their way out of an emotion. Thoughts in worry can be rational, analytic, rule-governed, and problem-solving. People with GAD tend to use worry thoughts to solve 'the problem of emotion.' Worry thinking does, in fact, help a little to calm emotions. But it doesn't work well or for long, because emotions are not 'problems' that needs to be solved. Uncomfortable emotions signal that there may be problems in getting your basic needs or goals met.

TABLE 8.3. Steps in Emotional Processing and Regulation Training

Step 1: Psychoeducation about emotions and rationale for training
>   Handout 8.4, About Emotion and Worry

Step 2: Techniques for evoking emotions and increasing emotional processing
>   Mindfulness
>   Empathic responding
>   Guided imagery
>   Focused exploration of the past
>   Empty chair
>   Letter writing
>   Narratives
>   Two-chair technique
>   Systematic evocation of feelings
>   Unhooking
>   Diaries of feelings

Step 3: Strategies for regulating emotions
>   Reducing emotional vulnerability
>   Increasing positive emotional events
>   Mindfulness
>   Taking opposite action
>   Distress tolerance techniques
>   Thinking of pros and cons
>   Distraction
>   Self-soothing
>   Improving the moment
>   Anger management

From *Treating Generalized Anxiety Disorder* by Jayne L. Rygh and William C. Sanderson. Copyright 2004 by The Guilford Press. Permission to photocopy this table is granted to purchasers of this book for personal use only (see copyright page for details).

"It is not clear why this pattern of excessive worry develops in some people. It may be due to a biological difference. Some people may have more exaggerated or intense emotions, and these interfere with their abilities to concentrate or to act in a collected manner when they are upset. People with GAD may have learned as children that emotions were dangerous, bad, or problematic, either for themselves or for others. Or they may have a history of unsatisfied basic needs, and so feel the natural negative emotional consequences of those unsatisfied needs—for example, a frequent and repeated state of internal distress. Or there may be a combination of these or other factors. Whatever the reason, we believe that some people with GAD will benefit from reconnecting with their emotional experience, for three reasons. First, reconnecting with your emotional experience helps you reconnect with your fundamental needs. Second, when you have reconnected with those needs, you can then find better ways to meet those needs. Third, this treatment will help you learn new and better ways to regulate the intensity of your emotions. The strategy of worry can still be used for times when problem solving can really help rather than hurt."

Handout 8.5 can then be given to the client to review these points.

ABOUT EMOTIONS AND WORRY

About Emotions

- Emotions include love, joy, anger, sadness, fear, anxiety, shame, and guilt.
- Emotions have useful purposes:
    1. They tell us and others about our basic needs.
    2. They motivate our actions.
- Actions motivated by emotions can be constructive, destructive, or neutral.

About Worry and Generalized Anxiety Disorder (GAD)

- Worry thoughts tend to be rational, analytic, rule-governed, and aimed at problem solving.
- Worry thoughts naturally suppress intense emotions.
- People with GAD see intense emotions as problems to be solved.
- People with GAD use worry thoughts to try to solve the problems of intense emotions. Doing this works a little bit, but not very well.

What Helps Worry in GAD?

- Understanding that an emotion is not a "problem." It cannot be rationally solved.
- Realizing that an emotion is, instead, an important signal that basic needs, concerns, or goals are (or are not) being met.
- Reconnecting with basic needs through deepening emotional experience.
- Learning better ways to get needs met.
- Learning better ways to manage intense or unpleasant emotions.

Step 2: Techniques for Evoking Emotions and Increasing Emotional Processing

A variety of techniques can be used to evoke and increase processing of emotional experience. See the middle section of Table 8.3 for an overview of the techniques we discuss here. All of these techniques increase awareness of emotions and provide exposures to these emotions. These exposures counteract experiential avoidance. The techniques include mindfulness, empathic responding, guided imagery, focused explorations of the past, the empty chair, letter writing, narratives, the two-chair technique, systematic evocation of feelings, unhooking, and diaries of feelings. Some of these techniques have been presented earlier in this book; we refer to these earlier discussions as each of the techniques is discussed below.

Since mindfulness training has been extensively described in the preceding section of this chapter, the reader is referred there for information on implementing this technique. In the context of emotional processing, mindfulness is helpful at increasing client awareness and identification of emotions, as well as practicing the ability to experience an emotion without acting on it.

Empathic responding has been briefly discussed in Chapter 2 as an important therapist factor in building and maintaining positive rapport. Here, it can be used as a therapist tool for increasing the client's awareness of and ability to describe and process emotional states. Newman et al. (2004) have suggested paying attention to markers of emotionality, such as changes in voice (pace, tone, volume) and changes in nonverbal behaviors (facial expression, posture, nonverbal utterances). When such markers are noted, the therapist can reflect what is believed to be the client's emotional state with comments such as "It sounds or looks like you are feeling [emotion]. Is that right?" The therapist can also inquire whether the client might be experiencing other emotions that would fit the situation or context of discussion, with questions such as "Do you notice any other feelings?" or "I wonder if there might be [another emotion]?" In addition, the therapist can simply ask the client to identify what he or she is feeling and ask the client to stay with that feeling. If a client suddenly disengages from a feeling (by changing topics or appearing to shut off emotionally), the therapist should inquire about the client's immediate experience. Often clients with GAD describe what they are thinking instead of feeling. When this occurs, the therapist can redirect the client not to use his or her head, but to speak "from the gut." Asking the client to focus on the sensations in his or her body often helps the client to connect or reconnect with feelings. It is important to note that this process is particularly helpful when the client is experiencing negative emotions in relation to the therapist. These instances can be uncomfortable; they require the therapist to sit through his or her own negative emotions in response. But it is important that the therapist not join the client in experiential avoidance at these times. Instead, the therapist should work to model acceptance and tolerance of the client's and his or her own negative emotions. This technique is further discussed in the following section, as an aspect of working through problems in the therapeutic relationship.

Imagery training is the same basic technique as that described in Chapter 5 as "positive imagery." It is a cognitive technique for altering physiological arousal with positive images. Here, the same type of training can be used to induce different emotional states for the purpose of clarifying and intensifying the emotional experience.

A focused exploration of the past has been presented as a schema therapy technique in Chapter 5. In Chapter 5, this technique has been described as a way to help the client gain a deeper understanding of the origins of his or her core beliefs. Here, the technique is a very effective tool for evoking and processing powerful emotional memories. It can be used to help the client identify the emotions that are evoked, and to identify and validate basic needs associated with those emotions.

Two other schema therapy techniques, the empty chair and letter writing, can be used as follow-ups to the prior technique to further explore and express any inhibited emotions. With these latter two techniques, the client is encouraged to express his or her feelings fully to an imagined other in an empty chair, or to do so by writing a letter. These are not intended as actual communications to be carried out in real-life settings. Instead, these techniques provide safe environments where the client can get in touch with inhibited emotions without any negative repercussions. In both exercises, the client is instructed to begin with the statement "I [emotion] you because . . . ". As Newman et al. (2004) have noted, the inhibited emotions may be positive (e.g., love), as well as negative.

Narratives can be used to evoke emotions associated with significant events in the client's life. They differ from focused explorations of the past in that narratives use detailed narratives of memories as the starting point, rather than bodily sensations to call up other associations with those sensations. In a narrative, the client is instructed to give vivid descriptions of everything in the memory (all external and internal stimuli). Again, the client is encouraged to sit with any feelings that are evoked.

The two-chair technique is used when conflicting or different emotions are present in relation to a situation or event. The client is asked to express one of these emotions fully as he or she sits in one chair, and then to express the other emotion fully while sitting in another chair. Throughout the exercise, the client is instructed to have each side try to convince the other side of the validity of that side and the actions that should be taken in accordance with that side. Through this process, all aspects of each emotional stance are fully explored.

When clients report that they are unaware of an emotional reaction, or that their reaction took them by surprise or confused them, the therapist should fully explore these instances. Newman et al. (2004) suggests using Greenberg's technique called "systematic evocation of feelings." This technique requires the client to imagine vividly, and in slow motion, the scene in which the "unknown" or "problematic" emotion occurred. Every detail of the scene, and of the client's feelings while inside the scene, is to be carefully described. Often clients begin to recognize subtle as well as more substantial emotional reactions with this technique.

Newman et al. (2004) present "unhooking" as a technique to be used by the therapist when it becomes apparent that he or she has become "hooked" into the client's pattern of avoidance. Indications of becoming hooked are when the therapist experiences the therapy as going nowhere or the relationship with the client as disconnected or emotionally detached, or when the therapist feels a sense of frustration or helplessness with the client. In such instances, the therapist must carefully attend to particulars of the session for places where he or she allowed the client to avoid emotional material (e.g., permitting the client to tell tangential stories, to provide irrelevant background, to change the focus of therapy, to provide only abstract or global information about events or feelings, or to engage the therapist in discussion of "why" the client or another has problems). The therapist must also increase awareness of his or her own vulnerabilities for getting hooked (e.g., discomfort with painful or other negative emotions, trying to get the client to feel better quickly rather than tolerate negative emotions). Unhooking involves purposefully redirecting the client to focus on emotional material at these times, rather than permitting avoidance.

Diaries of feelings can be used to self-monitor emotional states throughout the day or on a daily basis. The Emotion Log (see Handout 8.6) can be used for observing and describing emotions. The instructions for this log are similar to those for both versions of the Worry Episode Log (see Chapters 3 and 5), with the exception that the client is to self-monitor any emotional experience.

Step 3: Strategies for Regulating Emotions

Adaptive functioning requires individuals to modulate their emotions under certain circumstances. Individuals with GAD overutilize worry to decrease the intensity of emotions. It is therefore helpful to train clients to modulate their emotional experience with a variety of other strategies more appropriate than worry under certain circumstances. Linehan (1993a, 1993b) has presented five ways that the intensity and duration of emotions can be modulated. These include reducing one's vulnerability to emotional reactivity; increasing positive emotional events; applying mindfulness to current emotions; taking opposite actions; and utilizing distress tolerance techniques. Handout 8.7 covers these strategies for the client. In addition, for clients who exhibit anger control difficulties, an anger management strategy is presented; this strategy is taught as an alternative method for regulating emotional experience without suppressing or inhibiting it. The client can be given Handout 8.8 for managing anger.

Reducing vulnerability to emotional reactivity is an important first step in managing emotions. Factors that increase vulnerability to emotional reactivity are those that increase physical or environmental stress on the body. Poor diet and/or eating habits, inadequate sleep, inadequate self-care when ill, overloading one's daily schedule with obligations, and inadequate physical activity can all increase this vulnerability. Clients can take active steps to correct any of these factors. A client can alter eating habits by spacing meals at regular intervals and eating a nutritionally balanced diet in appropriately sized proportions. Sleep habits can be altered by setting regular bedtimes, restricting time in bed exclusively for sleep or sex, developing a regular relaxing routine before bed, and/or getting a consultation for medication if insomnia is chronic. Physical illnesses should be treated according to a doctor's recommendations. If possible, excessive amounts of obligatory activity should be examined for simplification or delegation. Physical condition can be improved with regular exercise.

The potential benefits of regular exercise are numerous. Regular exercise can operate as a buffer to stress. It can be used as a form of meditation or of exposure to internal sensations of physiological arousal. Regular exercise also possibly provides a way to increase flexibility in the autonomic nervous system and striate musculature. Despite these potential benefits, only one study (Martinsen, Sandvik, & Kolbjornsrud, 1989) could be found that suggested a positive outcome when exercise was used for clients with GAD. As such, this study offers only slight preliminary empirical support for the inclusion of exercise in a treatment package for GAD. Tkachuk and Martin (1999) have made several important recommendations for therapists who decide to include treatment recommendations for exercise. For therapists who do not have training in the principles of exercise physiology, liaisons with physicians and exercise physiologists are recom-

EMOTION LOG

Kinds of emotions: love, joy, anger, sadness, fear, anxiety, shame, guilt

Emotion rating scale

0	1	2	3	4	5	6	7	8
None		Low		Moderate		High		Extreme

Date	Identify emotion	Rate maximum intensity	Rate amount of control over emotion	Triggers	Mind (images, thoughts, assumptions, beliefs)	Body responses	Actions/behaviors

TIPS FOR MANAGING YOUR EMOTIONS

1. Reduce vulnerability through self-care (get sufficient food, sleep, exercise, etc.).

2. Do things that you enjoy. Schedule more activities you like.

3. Be mindful. Pay attention to the present. Turn your attention away from the past or future.

4. Take actions opposite to those urged by an emotion. For example, if you are feeling anxious or timid, stand erect, with your head up and shoulders back, with your mouth in a relaxed half-smile.

5. Help yourself tolerate distress through thinking of pros and cons (i.e., reviewing long-term costs and benefits), distraction, self-soothing, and improving the moment.

TIPS FOR MANAGING ANGER

1. Monitor your feelings of anger in daily life.

2. When a high level of anger is noticed, take a time out. Do not express the anger in action or word. Temporarily remove yourself from the situation (e.g., say, "Excuse me," or "Let me think about this and I'll get back to you," and leave).

3. During the time out, first identify what triggered the anger.

4. Once you have identified the trigger, identify your frustrated wants or needs.

5. Check for distortions in your interpretation of the trigger event.

6. Use diaphragmatic breathing or applied relaxation to calm arousal.

7. Try role reversal to increase empathy for the other person(s).

8. Explore options to get your wants and needs met, particularly assertive behaviors.

9. Do cost–benefit analyses of the various options.

10. When you are relatively calm, return to the situation and execute the best option.

mended to reduce the likelihood of possible ethical or legal conflicts. Prior to the initiation of any exercise program, the client should obtain medical clearance.

Several useful guidelines for prescribing exercise have been suggested by Sime (1996): identifying enjoyable exercise activities; exploring daily routines for exercise opportunities that serve functional purposes (e.g., walking or biking to work, doing chores around the home); making use of accessible facilities for exercise (e.g., public pools or lakes, fitness trails, exercise equipment); choosing enjoyable activities from a wide variety of choices; and exploring options for exercise within a positive social setting.

Increasing positive emotional events can be accomplished with the technique of pleasurable activity scheduling, presented in Chapter 7. The experience of positive emotion during these activities can be enhanced by practicing mindfulness (discussed earlier in this chapter) throughout engagement with each pleasurable activity.

"Taking opposite action" means to act in a way that is the opposite of or inconsistent with the emotion currently being experienced. The aim is not to block emotion with this technique; rather, it is to act in a way that is consistent with a different emotion. The idea is that the opposite action can then activate different emotional experiences. Here are some examples: If one is feeling fearful or anxious, the opposite action includes the overt behavior of approach, the posture of standing erect with head up and shoulders back, and a relaxed half-smiling facial expression; if the feeling is anger, the opposite action includes the overt behavior of sitting or standing back, the posture of standing off center with head down and shoulders slightly forward, and (again) a relaxed half-smiling facial expression.

Distress tolerance techniques are useful when it is important to tolerate negative emotions or the situations that evoke negative emotions. They include four strategies: thinking of pros and cons, distraction, self-soothing, and improving the moment. The middle two strategies can be problematic if they are used excessively to avoid emotional experience. However, they can be beneficial as temporary refuges from uncomfortable emotions when the benefits of tolerating particular situations outweigh the costs of avoiding.

Thinking of pros and cons is a way to determine the long-term costs and benefits of tolerating particular situations or emotions. The general strategy for conducting a cost–benefit analysis is presented in Chapter 5 and can be applied to tolerating any type of situation or negative emotion.

Distraction involves temporarily averting attention from stimuli that evoke negative emotions and turning attention toward other stimuli. Even though excessive worry is an example of an overuse of the distraction strategy, distraction can be valuable under certain circumstances. For example, Richard realized that it would be better to tolerate the distress he experienced at the playground with his daughter than to avoid the playground altogether (see Chapter 5). In this instance, Richard could use the distraction strategy by reading the paper, engaging in pleasant conversation with another parent, or planning his next vacation while his daughter played at the playground.

"Self-soothing" means comforting, nurturing, or being kind to oneself through any or all of the five senses (seeing, hearing, smelling, tasting, and touching) while tolerating negative emotions or difficult situations. To continue with the example above, Richard could attend to the beautiful weather, the sensations of the warm sun and air, pleasant breezes, the birds singing, and the lovely scenery at the park while his daughter played.

Improving the moment can be accomplished in several ways. One can stay mindful in the moment, find or create meaning for a negative emotional experience, turn to God for strength to withstand emotional distress, or use one of the relaxation techniques (progressive muscular relaxation [PMR], DB, or applied relaxation [AR]) presented in Chapter 6.

Clients with GAD may exhibit difficulties in regulating anger, particularly when they perceive their self-esteem or well-being as threatened. Such difficulties are apparent in clients who report frequent negative outcomes from altercations or angry outbursts with others. Clients can be taught the following steps to regulate anger (Handout 8.8 summarizes these for clients' use):

1. Clients should utilize mindfulness to monitor feelings in daily life.
2. When a client feels a high level of anger, he or she should take a time out. Instead of expressing the anger in action or word, the client should temporarily separate him- or herself from the situation (e.g., by saying, "Excuse me," or "Let me think about this and I'll get back to you," and leaving the situation).
3. In the time out, the client should first identify what triggered the anger.
4. The client should then identify the wants or needs he or she wishes to be met or addressed in the event or situation.
5. Next, the client should check for distortions in his or her interpretation of the trigger event. Examples include thoughts, assumptions, or beliefs that others are "wrong" or "unfair." Excessive anger is associated with distortions in these types of cognition. The cognitive restructuring (CR) exercises described in Chapter 5 can be used to recognize and challenge any distortions in these types of cognitions.
6. The client can use DB or AR to counter excess physiological arousal. (These techniques may also be used later during the confrontation with problematic situations.)
7. The client can also try role reversals (described in the next section). Role reversals may increase feelings of empathy for and awareness of the distorted perceptions of, others.
8. The client should explore possible options for trying to meet or fill wants or needs. In particular, he or she should identify assertive behaviors (again, see the next section) that permit confrontation of problematic situations and maximize the likelihood of obtaining objectives with respect, as opposed to overly aggressive behaviors that can damage relationships.
9. The client should do cost–benefit analyses (see Chapter 5) of expressing him- or herself at the height of emotion (these should include both short- and long-term consequences). These analyses can strengthen the client's resolve to contain behaviors that could create short-term benefit (feeling better) at the expense of long-term damage to a relationship.
10. When relatively calm, the client should return to the situation and execute an assertive response to confront the problematic situation and express needs, as opposed to executing overly aggressive behaviors that can damage relationships or passive behaviors that can maintain the problem.

The therapist can also suggest that the client identify events that are likely to evoke anger in the future. Imagery can be used to help the client prepare for such events.

INTERPERSONAL EFFECTIVENESS

Several lines of research (see Chapter 1) have indicated that interpersonal problems are related to poor outcomes in traditional CBT generally and in CBT for GAD in particular. Recurrent interpersonal problems are a key feature of personality disorders. Unfortunately, many interventions for these types of disorders have not undergone rigorous empirical scrutiny to determine effectiveness. (A notable exception is Linehan's [1993a, 1993b] dialectical behavior therapy for borderline personality disorder). In a continuing attempt to close this gap, Newman et al. (2004) have developed a treatment package for clients with GAD and interpersonal difficulties, which currently is being tested. Since definitive outcome research on effectiveness is not yet available, these techniques should be reserved for clients with interpersonal difficulties and should be used with this caution in mind.

Newman et al.'s treatment is an integrative therapy for GAD that incorporates interpersonal and emotional processing therapies with CBT. Many of their techniques for emotional processing have been included in the preceding section. Their techniques for treating interpersonal problems are discussed below. These researchers believe that the interpersonal patterns of those with GAD are associated with their excessive focus on anticipating threat and avoiding painful emotions. This focus interferes with their attending to and expressing personal needs and the needs of others within interpersonal situations. In efforts to avoid criticism and negative feelings, individuals with GAD often appear distant and cold. Ironically, this often results in others' becoming more critical and negative in relation to these individuals. Newman et al. suggest four treatment targets: problems in current relationships, developmental origins of current relationship problems, interpersonal problems within the client–therapist relationship, and avoidance of emotion. Basic CBT techniques of exposure, modeling, and skills training are used together with techniques drawn from interpersonal and emotional processing therapy models throughout this treatment. Many of these techniques are used to expose clients to feared emotions. The goal of treatment is to help these clients shift their focus of attention away from anticipating threat and avoiding emotions, and toward becoming more open and aware of their interpersonal needs, more vulnerable and spontaneous in the expression of those needs, and more empathetic in responding to others. In essence, a client is encouraged to develop awareness in relation to his or her own feelings and actions and those of others. In addition, the client is taught how he or she may behave differently.

Presenting the Rationale for Targeting Interpersonal Problems

When significant interpersonal problems are identified, the therapist explains how they can contribute to GAD and how treatment can help them.

> "We have reasons both to approach and to avoid interpersonal interactions. We approach interaction where we expect our needs to be met, and we avoid interaction where we expect pain or frustration of needs. Our expectations in relationships develop over time and are based on our experiences within earlier relationships. Once expectations develop, they become automatic—that is, they are no longer conscious. Once they are automatic, they result in habitual patterns of relating that may or may not work well within new relationships. At

times, we can find ourselves behaving in ways that recreate the old patterns, even though a new relationship is initially unlike the original ones.

"People with GAD tend toward patterns of interaction that are highly focused on avoiding pain and/or protecting themselves from potential pain. This focus interferes with their being open enough to recognize and express their own and others' needs within interactions. These kinds of patterns tend to be experienced by both them and the other people as frustrating and dissatisfying. These negative consequences spur those with GAD toward further avoidance and protection in interpersonal situations. Although avoidance and protection may be effective for relieving distress in the short term, they prevent needs from being expressed and met within relationships. This works to maintain dissatisfactions within relationships over the long term.

"Successful relationships require that we accept and tolerate emotional experience within us and others, even though it may be uncomfortable at times. If the interaction involves a problem in need of resolution, it is very important that we tolerate negative emotions while we attempt to locate the source of the problem. The source of an interpersonal problem may be in our old expectations (automatic thoughts, assumptions, and beliefs about relationships) and habitual patterns of relating. Or the problem may be in aspects of the present relationship that frustrate needs, cause pain, or a combination of both. Individuals with GAD often avoid fully experiencing their emotions, and this hampers them in locating sources of interpersonal problems. In addition, they are less able to recognize joy and other positive emotions in themselves and others. This tends to maintain negative expectations about relationships as well as the problematic patterns of interaction.

"This part of treatment will focus on helping you to recognize patterns of avoidance and protection within yourself and in your interactions with others. The techniques in this part of the treatment will help you to identify and clarify your emotions in relation to others, identify the basic needs that you want filled within those relationships, and identify and alter expectations and habitual patterns of behavior that prevent you from getting your needs met. You will learn and practice skills to increase the chances that others will be receptive to your needs. You will learn and practice techniques that help you to identify and clarify the needs of others as well. You will also learn and practice strategies for respectfully not filling others' needs, should you determine this not to be in your best interest. In addition, we will be exploring our therapeutic relationship to identify any patterns of avoidance and protection that may occur within our sessions. Although this may be temporarily uncomfortable for both of us, acknowledging problems that come up in our relationship will help us work out mutually agreeable solutions for keeping therapy on track.

"Throughout this treatment, I will be actively directing you to focus on your feelings. These can help you identify what you need and want in relation to another. You can then also better understand your behavior with others and the impact of these behaviors in the relationship. If you begin to experience my behavior as too frustrating or uncomfortable, and I do not seem to be aware of your level of discomfort, I want you to tell me. This is very important, because I can then adjust my behavior. I want to maintain a good working relationship with you through this sometimes difficult process. What's most important is that you maintain a solid feeling of safety with me. If at any time you do not feel safe, please let me know."

There are numerous techniques for bringing about change in interpersonal relationships (see Table 8.4). These techniques fall into two general categories. The first category consists of techniques that teach adaptive interpersonal behaviors. The second consists of techniques that raise awareness of problematic interpersonal patterns. Together, these interventions increase the client's awareness of emotional experiences within relationships and provide repeated opportunities to experience how conflicts generated by unmet needs can be resolved with newly acquired skills. These interventions allow the client to experience how openness, vulnerability, and spontaneity can lead to closeness in relationships.

Teaching Adaptive Behaviors

The techniques in this section educate the client about alternative sets of behavior that can be used in interpersonal situations. Assertiveness training teaches behaviors that maximize the probability of getting one's needs or wants met. Specific skills can also be taught for communicating empathy and maintaining self-respect within interactions. Role plays provide opportunities for modeling and practicing newly learned behaviors.

Assertiveness Training

Assertiveness training is appropriate for clients who exhibit difficulties in any of the following areas: difficulty in making reasonable requests of others or standing up for one's rights; problems with refusing unreasonable or unwanted requests (saying no); difficulty in adequately or appropriately resolving conflicts (e.g., backing down prematurely or using intimidation); and/or difficulty in being heard by others and having one's points of view taken into consideration. Individuals who have difficulties asserting themselves tend to exhibit two extremes of behavior in relation to trying to obtain objectives: They tend to be either excessively passive (respectful of others and not respectful of themselves) or excessively aggressive (disrespectful of others and respectful of them-

---

TABLE 8.4. Interventions for Interpersonal Problems

Teaching adaptive behaviors
- Assertiveness training
- Skills for communicating empathy and self-respect
- Role plays

Raising awareness of problematic patterns
- Reversed role plays
- Reframing the relationship
- Addressing in-session behaviors
- Exploring links of present with past
- Addressing alliance ruptures

From *Treating Generalized Anxiety Disorder* by Jayne L. Rygh and William C. Sanderson. Copyright 2004 by The Guilford Press. Permission to photocopy this table is granted to purchasers of this book for personal use only (see copyright page for details).

selves). The ultimate goal of assertiveness training is to teach clients how to maintain respectful attitudes and behaviors toward both themselves and others in their attempts to obtain needs and wants. Assertiveness training consists of two steps. The first is to help clients identify their personal objectives; the second is to teach behaviors that maximize chances for obtaining those objectives. Handout 8.9 summarizes these skills for clients.

Individuals who have difficulties asserting themselves sometimes have trouble saying what they want or need in specific situations. These clients may exhibit reticence when directly asked what they want, and may readily minimize or dismiss any identified needs as unimportant. Under such circumstances, the therapist may need to ask questions and listen for frustration, irritation, resentment, or anger in relation to others. The therapist can point out that negative emotions are a natural consequence when wants and needs are frustrated. Negative emotions can be useful for identifying important unmet needs and wants.

When personal objectives are identified, some clients exhibit excessive anxiety, guilt, or anger. They may assume that others will respond negatively (with rejection, anger, or hurt) if they assert themselves. CR exercises (see Chapter 5) may be required to recognize distortions and alter these assumptions.

Once the client's personal objectives are identified, the following points (see Handout 8.9) will maximize the clear expression of wants and needs and the probability of positive responses from others:

- The client should use "I" statements when expressing wants and needs (e.g., "I want" vs. "You should").
- Wants or needs should be expressed in concrete terms (e.g., specific behaviors, specific schedules, etc.), rather than in general terms (e.g., characteristics of other, general labels, etc.). Example: "I want to get together more frequently, like once a week" versus "I want you to be less self-centered."
- The client should state the positive consequences for the emotional condition of the relationship if the other responds to the client's wants and needs. Example: "I will feel a lot happier with you and better about our relationship if we are spending more time together."

If the interaction involves addressing problematic behavior in another, the assertion should include the following points:

- Again, the client should use "I" statements to express his or her feelings in relation to the other's behavior. Example: "I feel upset" versus "You make me so angry."
- The problem should be identified in concrete behavioral terms, rather than in global statements about the other. Example: "I feel upset when you arrive an hour late and have not called to explain the reason" versus "You're such an inconsiderate person."
- The negative consequences of the behavior for the relationship should be expressed. Example: "I was worried that something bad had happened to you. Seeing that you're fine makes me wonder if you care about me and our relationship."
- The client should state wants and needs by following the points in the preceding set of instructions. Example: "I want you to call me when you are going to be late. Calling commu-

ASSERTIVENESS SKILLS

Identify Personal Objectives

- Negative emotions indicate unmet wants or needs.
- Conduct cognitive restructuring to reduce excessive anxiety, guilt, or anger over personal objectives.

Increase clarity of expression

How to express yourself:
- Keep your voice calm (use relaxation techniques if necessary).
- Make eye contact.
- Stand or sit erect and face the other.
- Maintain the focus on your objective.
- Do not respond to attacks; do not be diverted from your objective.
- Be a "broken record," repeating your position until the other responds.

What to say:

If objective is to gain something positive:

1. Use "I" statements to express what you want or need.
2. Express your want or need in concrete terms (state specific behaviors, rather than using general labels).
3. Express positive consequences for the relationship if the want or need is met.
4. Be prepared to negotiate something mutually agreeable.

If objective is to solve a problem:

1. Use "I" statements to express your feelings about the problem (e.g., "I feel disappointed, hurt, annoyed").
2. State the problem in concrete terms (again, speak about specific behaviors, rather than making global statements about the other).
3. Express negative consequences of the problem for the relationship.
4. Say what you want or need with "I" statements, being concrete and specific.
5. Be prepared to negotiate a mutually agreeable solution or to ask for suggestions for resolution.

nicates that you are concerned about my feelings and that you respect my time. If you do this, I'll remain happy to see you, even though you're late."

When making assertions, the client should stand up straight, look directly at the other, and speak in a calm voice (using relaxation techniques if necessary). The focus should be kept on the client's objectives throughout the assertion, and the client should refrain from responding to diversions or attacks. The "broken record" technique (repeating one's position or refusals until the other responds to the position or backs off) may be used if necessary. The client should prepare to negotiate mutually agreeable terms for resolution of the problem or ask for suggestions for resolution, when either is appropriate.

In instances where the assertion is appropriate for the situation and changes have not occurred over the course of time, the client should consider repeating the assertion. He or she should also consider making a realistic evaluation of the other's capability or desire to respond to the client's wants and needs. For example, the other's lack of resources or personal limitations, or excessive or inappropriate client wants or needs, indicate that other avenues for obtaining these objectives may need to be explored. Other possibilities may also need to be investigated in situations where the other is in a position of power over the client (e.g., the client's boss or parent) and where there is a history of abuse of power (i.e., the other arbitrarily exercises power regardless of what is reasonable, fair, or respectful). In such instances, the most appropriate assertive behavior may be for the client to work toward limiting or removing the power of the other over him or her (e.g., finding a new job, identifying points of leverage for changing the relationship, limiting time with a parent, or limiting financial controls).

On occasion, the other person will respond negatively despite an appropriate assertion. It is important to clarify for the client that the success or failure of an assertion is not dependent upon whether or not the other gives the client what he or she wants, or whether the other has a positive or negative response to the assertion. A successful outcome of behaving assertively is dependent upon whether or not the assertion is made in a way that is respectful and caring of both the self and the other. The following discussion covers behaviors that can be executed to maintain an empathic attitude and self-respect in interactions that are emotionally difficult.

Skills for Communicating Empathy and Self-Respect

Problems with maintaining empathy and self-respect are likely to occur when the client's interaction with another is driven by fear of not getting what he or she wants from the interaction. When this fear results in fight behaviors, empathy fails. The person may be aggressively self-protective, rather than receptive and open to the other. When the fear results in flight or freeze behaviors, the person may be overly passive and accommodating and may surrender self-respect. When either of these tendencies is acted out, communications with the other are disrupted. The client can be taught specific behaviors for communicating empathy and self-respect in emotionally difficult interpersonal situations.

Empathy Skills to Counteract a Fight Mode. When the fear activates fight responses, behaviors can include defensive statements, judgmental statements, angry silences, attacks, or threats.

These behaviors result in the other's feeling misunderstood and/or disrespected in the interaction. The other usually withdraws or fights back, as further attempts at communication are considered useless. When these fear-driven behaviors occur, it is important to point out to the client that these behaviors push others away. This will make it very difficult, if not impossible, for the client to get what he or she wants from the interaction. This is usually the opposite of what is intended. The client can be trained to execute a different set of behaviors at these times—empathic behaviors. Practice of empathic behaviors frequently results in the client feeling more empathic toward the other. Empathy for another can be communicated through the following (which are summarized for the client in Handout 8.10):

- The client should listen carefully for the feeling and content of the other's communication, without interrupting the other's communication.
- While listening, the client should demonstrate a respectful and open attitude even if he or she strongly disagrees with that view (i.e., judging, threatening, attacking, and/or responding defensively should be avoided). Being courteous (exercising self-control and self-discipline) and staying positive (demonstrating a pleasant demeanor) are essential throughout.
- The client's understanding of the other's communication should be reflected in efforts to identify the other's feeling and the content of the communication. The client can use statements such as this: "Let me see if I understand what you are saying. It sounds like you're feeling [emotion], because [reflection of content]."
- The client should then run an immediate check with the other as to whether this understanding is correct. Statements such as "Did I understand correctly?", "Did I get it?", or "Is that right?" are helpful.
- The client can ask for clarifications of any misunderstandings with statements such as "What part did I misunderstand?"

These points should be repeated until the other fully acknowledges that his or her communication has been correctly received. Then the client should proceed with the following:

- The client should look for the grains of truth in the other's communication, but should prepare to validate only those parts with which he or she can honestly agree. The other points should not be mentioned at this time.
- If the emotion (not necessarily the intensity of the emotional expression) experienced by the other makes sense in relation to the other's interpretation (even though the client may not agree with that interpretation) the client should prepare to validate the emotion. The intensity of the expression should not be mentioned at this time.
- The client can use statements such as this: "Yes, [restating those points with which the client can agree]. I understand how you would feel [emotion] in relation to [restating those points again]."

These types of statements communicate the client's awareness and understanding of the other's experience. Once the other feels that he or she is being respectfully heard and understood, he or she is more likely to be open to the client's assertions regarding other points of the matter.

HOW TO COMMUNICATE EMPATHY

Step 1: Listen.

How?

- Do not interrupt.
- Listen for both feeling and content in what the other says.
- Be respectful, courteous, and pleasant, even if you disagree.
- When the other has finished speaking, move to Step 2.

Step 2: Say what you think the other feels and has just said.

How?

- "Let me see if I understand what you're saying. It sounds like you are feeling [emotion] because [content]. Is that right?"
- If the other says that you do not yet understand, ask for further explanation. Repeat Steps 1 and 2 above.
- If the other says that you have it right, move to Step 3.

Step 3: Validate how the other person feels given how the other sees the situation.

How?

- Look for grains of truth in the other's interpretation. Agree with those parts without commenting on the other parts. "I can understand how you might think that [restate the other's interpretation] from [acknowledge the grains of truth]."
- When an emotion connected to a particular interpretation makes sense, validate that relationship. Refrain from commenting on the intensity of the emotion. "I also can understand how you would feel [emotion], given [restate the other's interpretation of the situation]."After completing these 3 steps, this point, you can say how you feel and how you see the situation, using assertiveness skills.

Maintaining Self-Respect in Communications. When fear activates freeze and/or flight responses, failures in maintaining self-respect occur. These behaviors include overly accommodating, apologetic, or self-demeaning statements or behaviors. These behaviors interfere with clear communications of the client's wants or needs. As a result, the other is less likely to recognize or feel responsible for attending to those wants or needs. When the flight mode of behavior is activated, the client can be trained to execute behaviors for maintaining self-respect in interactions. Execution of these behaviors often results in feelings of increased self-esteem. These behaviors are as follows (see Handout 8.11):

- The client should act and speak in ways that are consistent with personal morals and values.
- No apologies should be offered for differences of opinion or for things that are not the client's responsibility.
- Requests for unnecessary help or reassurance should be avoided.
- The client should not brush away compliments, but should simply smile and thank the complimenter.

Role Plays

In addition to learning basic skills for communicating assertively, empathically, and with self-respect, the therapist can model and have the client begin practicing these new behaviors through role plays. Role plays can be carried out in session with the therapist, can be done in the client's imagination, and/or can be assigned for practice in real life. Role plays that are conducted in imagination or in session with the therapist are particularly helpful and may be a necessary first step when the client is reporting high levels of anxiety about executing these behaviors with others. If the client is struggling with finding words or actions in playing the new role, the therapist can model various options and then ask the client to try them out. It is important to tell the client that feeling uncomfortable or like a "fraud" is to be expected when trying out these new roles. With repeated practice, the discomfort will lessen, and the roles will feel increasingly more natural and familiar.

Raising Awareness of Problematic Patterns

Problematic interpersonal patterns in clients with GAD result from their general tendencies to avoid emotional experience and to overutilize coping strategies that protect them against actual or potential pain. These interpersonal patterns interfere with the necessary openness and vulnerability for interpersonal connection.

A therapist can become aware of a client's avoidance of emotional experience when the therapist notices that he or she is behaving in ways that confirm or maintain the client's problematic patterns. As noted earlier in this chapter, Newman et al. (2004) describe this as becoming "hooked." A strong indication that the therapist has become "hooked" is a feeling that therapy is not progressing. The therapist may notice that he or she is bored or feels disconnected with the client in sessions. Or the therapist may notice that the client's communications are repeatedly

TIPS FOR MAINTAINING SELF-RESPECT IN COMMUNICATION

Be aware of your own morals and values. Act and speak in ways that are consistent with these. In addition, follow these suggestions:

1. Do not apologize for differences of opinion.
2. Do not apologize for things that are not your responsibility.
3. Do not ask for unnecessary help or reassurance.
4. Do not brush away compliments. Simply smile and say, "Thank you."

about others or off topic. The therapist may notice a feeling of apprehension about pursuing certain topics with the client. When any of these things occur, the treatment goal is to gently help the client "unhook" from this pattern by refocusing the client on his or her emotional experience with another inside and/or outside the therapy relationship. Newman et al. (2004) have described three general ways in which the therapist can use relationships to bring about change in interpersonal patterns. One way is to directly address various behaviors in the client that are contributing to problematic interactions. A second way is to link the client's interpersonal patterns with patterns in other (current and past) relationships. A third way is to explore phenomena in the therapeutic relationship, such as alliance ruptures. The process of "unhooking" the client from problematic patterns increases the client's awareness of underlying wants and needs that are motivating behavior and of specific maladaptive behaviors that are being used to meet those wants and needs. Once these things are brought into awareness, alternative behavioral strategies for meeting wants and needs can be practiced.

Numerous specific methods can be used to address a client's maladaptive interpersonal patterns. One method is to engage in reversed role plays with the client. Another method is for the therapist to mentally reframe the client's relationships as if the therapist is the other party in interactions with the client. A third is to comment on specific behaviors as they present themselves within the therapy relationship, in sessions. A fourth is to explore links between the client's present interpersonal patterns and those in the past. The last is to address ruptures in the therapeutic alliance. These methods not only increase the client's awareness of and responsibility for his or her contributions to problematic interactions, but provide positive interpersonal experiences with maintaining vulnerability, openness, and spontaneity in relationships. Each of these methods is described in detail below.

Reversed Role Plays

Reversed role plays can be used to increase a client's awareness of the effects of his or her behavior on others, as well as to increase the client's empathy for others in interactions. In reversed role plays, the client is instructed to perceive the situation as if he or she stepped inside the other's shoes and is looking and talking back to the client. The therapist acts out the way the client talks and acts in the interaction. Sometimes a client will try to use the exercise to further validate his or her position. To counteract this tendency, the therapist should state clearly that the client is to suspend his or her own perspective temporarily, and fully embrace the role and perspective of the other in the interaction throughout the exercise. The client should be instructed to pay attention to what he or she feels and thinks in response to the therapist's role during the reversed role play. The therapist can explain that the purpose of the role reversal is to give the client a firsthand experience of what it is like to interact with him- or herself.

Reframing the Relationship

"Reframing the relationship" involves perceiving the client's behaviors from the perspective of the other person in the client's daily life, and reflecting likely feelings and thoughts of the other in relation to the client's statements and behaviors. This method requires the therapist to imagine him- or herself as the other person interacting with the client as the client gives a blow-by-blow description of a problematic interaction. The therapist must pay careful attention to his or her feelings and thoughts in relation to the client from this perspective. These feelings can then be presented to the client in an open and nonjudgmental atmosphere. The following clinical vignette demonstrates this process. (Once more, the client is Richard.)

CLIENT: I had a fight with my wife and kids last weekend that I feel bad about.

THERAPIST: What happened?

CLIENT: I wanted to go for a hike because I'm cooped up indoors all week at work. I thought it would be good for the whole family to get some exercise and fresh air, so I tried to get them to go with me. We ended up getting into an argument and then I went in to work instead. I don't know what happened. I'm trying to spend more time with them, but this didn't work. It was bad.

THERAPIST: OK. Let's take this situation apart. I want you to give me a blow-by-blow account of the whole conversation between you, your wife, and your kids. I want you to tell me the exact wording of what everyone said, and I want you to describe the exact actions of everyone involved. How did it start?

CLIENT: I said, "How about going to the state park to take a hike?" My wife made a funny face and said, "I don't really want to do that." She said, "Let's go to see that new Disney movie with the kids." She said, "The kids have been asking to see it all week." She said that Janis—Janis is her friend—said it was good, and said, "Janis's husband liked it." At that point my kids started shrieking and jumping up and down, saying, "Say yes, Daddy."

THERAPIST: And then what happened?

CLIENT: I didn't say anything. I smiled at my kids, but I wasn't happy.

THERAPIST: Then what happened?

CLIENT: My wife started looking up the movie schedule with the kids.

THERAPIST: And what did you do?

CLIENT: I went out to the garage and started cleaning it for about an hour and a half.

THERAPIST: Then what?

CLIENT: We ate lunch, and while we were eating, I started complaining about my work.

THERAPIST: What exactly did you say?

CLIENT: I was saying, "I feel stressed out about one of my cases." I was saying, "I don't know if I should go to the movies. I have a lot of work."

THERAPIST: And?

CLIENT: My wife got really mad. She said, "You're always working. Why can't you make any time for us?" She said, "I thought you were working on this in therapy."

THERAPIST: And what did you say?

CLIENT: I yelled at her. I said, "What do you want from me? I've been here all morning, haven't I?" Then she yelled back, "You're not here. First you're working in the garage, and now your mind is on your job."

THERAPIST: What did you say?

CLIENT: I said, "You don't appreciate anything that I do," and I left the room. Then, about a half hour later, she announced they were leaving and asked if I was coming along, in this angry voice. I said "No!" angrily, and then I went to work.

THERAPIST: As you've been describing this interaction, I've been imaging myself as if I were your wife—hearing your statements and experiencing your actions. I noticed that I started feeling confused, then frustrated and angry, and thinking that you do not view family time as important. Do you think that that is what she was feeling and thinking?

CLIENT: Well, she said that and expressed those feelings, but how could she feel or think that? I was trying to spend time with them. I wanted to be with them. I just wanted to be outside and do something that involved exercise.

THERAPIST: Thinking back to what you said, do you think that you expressed that clearly?

CLIENT: Well, no. I guess I just asked if they wanted to go on a hike.

THERAPIST: Is there a reason why you didn't express what you wanted more clearly?

CLIENT: I was afraid they wouldn't want to go because it's a so-so activity for my wife. I was afraid she wouldn't want to do this with me.

THERAPIST: And when she confirmed that she wasn't crazy about the idea and presented another one that your kids liked, then what?

CLIENT: Then I really felt like I couldn't say anything, because I was afraid my kids would be mad and be disappointed if we did what I wanted.

THERAPIST: Do you remember what you did?

CLIENT: I smiled.

THERAPIST: And then?

CLIENT: I went out to the garage to work.

THERAPIST: As your therapist, I am hearing your fear of rejection in your tentative request, and your avoidance of emotional discomfort by smiling at your kids and then leaving the situation to work. Do you think your wife or your kids knew you didn't like this idea and wanted to do something else?

CLIENT: No. I guess what I did was confusing.

THERAPIST: How do you think you could have expressed yourself more clearly?

CLIENT: I don't know.

THERAPIST: Think about some of the assertiveness and empathy skills you learned last week and how you might apply them here.

CLIENT: OK. I could have said, "I want to do something fun with everyone today. I'm really tired of sitting indoors all week, so I want to do something outside that involves exercise. How about hiking at the park?"

THERAPIST: I just imagined hearing that, and I had a completely different emotional response to you. It felt good, because it sounded like you want to spend time with us and you want to find an activity that we all will enjoy. If I didn't want to go on a hike, I would know to think of alternative activities that are outside and involve exercise. I wouldn't even consider a movie with that information.

CLIENT: Things probably would have turned out differently if I had said that. I probably would have had a good time with my family instead of overworking again.

THERAPIST: Right. It's hard to be open and vulnerable with others about what you want when you're afraid—but if you express what you want clearly, with care and respect for yourself and others, you'll recognize that you're more likely to get what you want.

Addressing In-Session Behaviors

When the therapist directly experiences specific in-session problematic behaviors that contribute to the client's interpersonal problems, Newman et al. (2004) suggests that the therapist clearly state in an open, empathic, and nondefensive manner how these behaviors affect the way the therapist feels in the relationship with the client. For example, the therapist might say in response to the client's changing the topic, "When you change the topic, I feel like you are pushing me away." Or he or she might say in response to the client's not answering a question, "When you don't answer my question, I feel like you are telling me that my questions are unimportant." Or when a client is speaking rapidly without pause, the therapist might comment, "When you speak so rapidly without pausing, I feel like you are not interested in what I might have to say." These assertions should be followed with asking the client how he or she feels in relation to the therapist's statement. If a client tries to justify his or her behavior by saying, "I did that because I was uncomfortable," it is important for the therapist to stress that this justification does not take away the effect of these behaviors. The therapist can state, "I understand your discomfort, but that does not diminish how this behavior affects me." This process helps the client become more cognizant of responsibility for the effect of his or her behavior on others.

Exploring Links of Present with Past

Linking patterns in current relationships with patterns in past relationships helps to increase the client's awareness of the current patterns and to identify their origins, as well as the underlying beliefs or schemas that generate these patterns. When describing a current problematic interaction, clients often spontaneously report other interpersonal situations where they have noticed similar feelings and patterns of interaction. A therapist can further assist a client in linking present with past experiences by encouraging the client to focus on the feelings experienced within these interactions and to report any images or associations to these feelings. The therapist can then ask the client to trace the feelings back to the first time that he or she became aware of these feelings. When early memories surface that indicate the primary relationship where the pattern developed, the therapist and client can fully explore these memories. The memories should be examined for how the interaction contributed to the development of the client's beliefs about relationships, fears in relationships, and avoidant and protective coping strategies as useful adaptations for that particular interpersonal situation. The beliefs, fears, and coping strategies can then be examined for their adaptive value in relation to the current interpersonal situation that initially evoked these feelings and patterns of interaction. The following clinical vignette illustrates this process.

THERAPIST: Do you recall the feelings that you had before you started to argue with your wife?

CLIENT: Yes. I remember feeling both anxious and irritated.

THERAPIST: I want you to close your eyes and try to imagine yourself in that situation again. As if it was happening right now.

CLIENT: OK.

THERAPIST: Are you able to feel like you're there again?

CLIENT: Yes. I'm feeling anxious and irritated.

THERAPIST: Where are you feeling this in your body?

CLIENT: In my chest and throat. There's tightness.

THERAPIST: Focus on these feelings in your body. Let your mind float to other times when you had these same feelings. Let your mind float back to the first time you noticed these feelings in your body. Tell me what's happening in any images that come to mind.

CLIENT: (*Pause*) . . . I'm young and wanting to play outside. I ask my mom if I can go out, but she's telling me to go upstairs and clean my room.

THERAPIST: How old are you?

CLIENT: I'm about 5.

THERAPIST: Try to stay with this image. . . . Let yourself be 5-year-old Richard who wants to go outside. . . . Let yourself feel like 5-year-old Richard . . . noticing what little Richard is feeling . . . noticing what little Richard is doing and saying. . . . Let me hear you as you ask your mom to go outside.

CLIENT: Mommy, can I go outside?

THERAPIST: Let me know what you are feeling as you ask your mommy. . . .

CLIENT: I'm feeling excited because I see my friends playing in the yard next door.

THERAPIST: What is your mother doing and saying? . . . What is little Richard feeling in relation to his mother? . . .

CLIENT: She's ironing my dad's shirts, and she's looking down with a stern expression, not happy. She's not looking at me. She's looking at her work. She tells me to go to my room to clean it.

THERAPIST: What are you feeling as she says this?

CLIENT: I'm feeling upset. I feel like I'm going to miss the fun. I feel like she didn't hear me.

THERAPIST: What are you saying or doing? Let me hear it. Describe it to me.

CLIENT: No, Mommy, I want to go outside (*in a voice of protest*). Jimmy's outside. I want to play.

THERAPIST: And what's happening?

CLIENT: She puts the iron down hard and looks at me with an angry expression. She tells me in a very harsh voice to go upstairs and clean my room.

THERAPIST: Keep going. . . . What are you feeling?

CLIENT: I'm really mad. I'm screaming, "No! I want to go outside!!" She's walking over to me, and she grabs my arm and face. It hurts. She's making me look into her eyes. I'm seeing this horrible face. It's this horrible face that I've never seen before. It's like she's become someone else and she's going to kill me if I say another word. I'm feeling really scared. She says very harshly, "I said, go to your room and clean it! You're going to stay in all day for talking back to me!!" I'm feeling terrible: sad, mad, and scared. I want to go outside, but I feel like that doesn't matter. I have to go work and have no fun to not see that face again. I feel like I can't say anything. It will only get worse if I talk back. (*Richard suddenly opens his eyes as if he's now awake and states to the therapist:*)

That's when this pattern started. This type of interaction happened again in elementary school with that friend I horsed around with in school. Again, I got this harsh and unreasonable punishment for having fun. It's like I'm not entitled to enjoy my life.

THERAPIST: Let's look at the situation with your wife again. How did these beliefs and your behavior repeat this for you?

CLIENT: I wasn't comfortable telling everyone what I wanted, so I tried to let my wife know in a very indirect way. When I saw her face of displeasure—her face wasn't as bad as my mom's, though—I was seeing it as a confirmation of this belief that I'm not entitled to have fun with others.

THERAPIST: And what about your behavior?

CLIENT: I didn't say anything, because I thought it could only make matters worse. It was as if I felt that I didn't have the right to express myself to her or my kids, and if I did, something terrible would happen.

THERAPIST: Right. But what did you realize from our other exercise?

CLIENT: I have to express myself clearly to get what I want. My wife certainly is not my mom. I know my wife would have listened to me and cared about my happiness if I had been clear with her. My fear of being open and vulnerable with her doesn't fit.

THERAPIST: Right. But the only way to diminish this fear is to repeatedly be assertive with her and with others who are able to be concerned about your needs. In time, you will build up more and more experiences and become more emotionally convinced that these behaviors are safe and can lead to closer and more satisfying relationships.

One final note: It is important that these explorations not be used to avoid negative emotions that arise within the therapeutic relationship. Next, we address how to deal with ruptures in the therapeutic relationship due to negative feelings within the therapeutic interaction.

Addressing Alliance Ruptures

Dealing with alliance ruptures can be difficult for a therapist, because it means that the therapist must model openness, spontaneity, and vulnerability with the client in the here-and-now of the session when the client is experiencing negative emotions (anger, hurt, anxiety, or disappointment) toward the therapist or therapy. When a therapist avoids addressing an alliance rupture within the therapeutic relationship, the therapist is actively participating in—that is, remaining "hooked" into—the client's negative pattern of interaction. Directly addressing alliance ruptures is a way to "unhook" from these negative patterns. To "unhook" effectively, the therapist must be willing to expose him- or herself to negative emotional experience. If the therapist finds that he or she is avoiding talking about these ruptures with the client, the therapist should check whether he or she is engaging in experiential avoidance due to his or her own discomfort with expressions of anger, anxiety, disappointment, or pain. The most negative outcome of continued avoidance by the therapist is that the client abruptly terminates therapy without any previous discussion of problems.

It is not therapeutically helpful or productive for the therapist to assign responsibility for an alliance rupture to the client. Rather, the therapist must adopt an empathic attitude with the client even when the client's emotional reactions seem unreasonable or unfair. The therapist should look for and validate the grain of truth in whatever the client expresses, and should assume responsibility for any of his or her contributions to the client's negative feelings. Again, the therapist's role is to model openness, spontaneity, and vulnerability with the client even when the client's emotional experience is negative. This way of dealing with a rupture in a relationship provides the client with an interpersonal experience where openness, spontaneity, and vulnerability lead to a positive outcome—namely, greater closeness in the relationship. The method for dealing with alliance ruptures can be summarized in the following steps:

1. The therapist clearly communicates that he or she has noticed the client's statement or behavior, and invites the client to talk about it. Example: "I noticed that you have come late to our last two sessions. I'm wondering if there is something about me or our sessions that is bothering you."
2. The therapist reflects the client's feelings and perceptions, and checks whether or not the therapist's understanding is correct. Example: "It sounds like you've been feeling annoyed with me. When I repeatedly say, 'Do you know what I mean?' in our sessions, you're feeling like I'm expressing impatience with you and your progress. You're feeling like I'm saying you should be doing better by now. Is that right?"
3. The therapist finds the grain of truth in the client's statements, and validates his or her contribution to the negative interaction. Example: "I can see how you would feel bad about coming to see me if you are hearing this question as 'Haven't you gotten this yet?' I probably wouldn't want to come either if I were you. I appreciate your openness with letting me know how this question sounds and feels to you. I'm realizing right now that I ask that question very frequently with all of my clients. In my mind, when I ask that question, I'm wondering whether or not I've been clear in making my point. Thank you for making me aware of the negative effect of repeatedly asking this question."

TIME MANAGEMENT

Clients with GAD may experience undue stress from mismanagement of time. This occurs when they overextend themselves by taking on too many responsibilities, underestimate the time required to complete activities, or do not prioritize the relative importance of activities in terms of their personal values and life goals. Time management teaches clients how to prioritize activities according to values and life goals, and how to function more efficiently and effectively within specific time frames. The outcome of successful time management is a reduction in overall levels of stress. The following procedures are based on Craske, Barlow, and O'Leary (1992) and Roemer and Orsillo (2002), and are summarized in Handout 8.12. A client can be taught the following steps for managing time:

1. The client begins by identifying and/or clarifying his or her values and life goals.
2. The client then writes down all the activities that he or she feels need to be completed in the present, the near future, and the distant future.
3. The client separates all of these activities into two lists. One list is for the activities that are in line with the client's personal values and life goals. The other list is for all other activities.
4. The client focuses on the list of activities that are consistent with personal values and goals, and continues with Steps 5–8. The other list is set aside for Step 9.
5. The client organizes activities into the following categories: (A) ones that must be completed that day; (B) ones that need to be completed within the next 2–3 days; (C) activities that need to be completed within the same week; and (D) activities that can be completed at some later time.
6. The client estimates the amount of time required to complete each of the listed activities. If the client tends to chronically underestimate completion times, these estimates should be doubled, as a general rule.
7. The client enters the categorized activities on a weekly/monthly desk planner. Activities are scheduled within specific time frames. (If it is not possible for a client to structure activities according to times of the day—e.g., the client's work requires him or her to be on call—the therapist and client should discuss an alternative method for completing items within each day or week.) If there are too many activities for the allotted times, the client should reprioritize and/or redistribute the activities according to level of importance.
8. If there are opportunities or requests to take on additional obligations or responsibilities, the client should politely turn down (see "Assertiveness Skills") activities that do not comfortably fit within the planner, or should again reprioritize and redistribute existing activities.
9. The client uses assertiveness skills to delegate or discontinue the activities he or she has turned down.

TIPS FOR MANAGEMENT OF TIME

1. Identify and/or clarify your personal values and life goals.

2. Write down all activities that need to be completed in the present, the near future, and the distant future.

3. Separate activities into two lists: activities in line with your personal values and life goals, and all other activities.

4. Take the first list and continue with Steps 5–8. Set aside the second list for Step 9.

5. Categorize each activity according to level of priority: (A) activities that must be completed that day; (2) activities that must be completed within the next 2–3 days; (C) activities that must be completed that week; (D) activities that can be completed at a later time.

6. Estimate the time required to complete each activity. If you tend to underestimate completion times, double the estimates.

7. On a weekly/monthly desk planner, schedule the activities in the A, B, and C categories. (If it is not possible to schedule activities at specific times—e.g., an on-call work schedule—discuss alternative methods for scheduling with your therapist.) If there are too many activities for allotted times, reprioritize and/or redistribute activities according to level of importance.

8. Check your planner before accepting additional responsibilities. Either politely turn down activities that do not comfortably fit within your planner, or (again) reprioritize and redistribute existing activities.

9. Delegate or discontinue the activities you have turned down. Use assertiveness skills as needed.

Note. Based on Craske, Barlow, and O'Leary (1992) and Roemer and Orsillo (2002).

CHAPTER NINE

Ending Treatment

Before ending treatment, the therapist must determine the client's readiness for termination. In making this determination, the therapist must consider whether all relevant techniques have been presented to, and sufficiently mastered by, the client. If so, the therapist then must determine whether or not the techniques have proven to be effective in reducing the frequency, intensity, and duration of worry. Effectiveness of the treatment can be assessed with the methods presented in Chapter 3 (interviews and questionnaires), as well as from the client's spontaneous statements.

When treatment has not been sufficiently effective, the therapist and client will need to identify impediments to progress and explore further treatment options (such as techniques for addressing interpersonal problems or emotional avoidance, medication, etc.) accordingly. In Richard's case, it became apparent by midtreatment that some of the triggers for his worry episodes at work were related to his interactions with certain colleagues. Upon further assessment of these interactions, it became apparent that Richard's patterns of interaction with these individuals contributed to problems in these relationships. The negative outcomes of these interpersonal patterns exacerbated and maintained some of his worry. Additional techniques to increase Richard's awareness of his contributions to these problems and to help him alter his patterns of interaction with these individuals significantly improved these relationships and significantly reduced the worry associated with the prior problems. By the conclusion of treatment, Richard's posttreatment questionnaires and his self-report indicated significant improvement. As noted at the end of Chapter 3, his scores on the self-report assessments at posttreatment were as follows: Beck Anxiety Inventory, 10; Beck Depression Inventory—II, 7; Penn State Worry Questionnaire, 45; and Generalized Anxiety Disorder Questionnaire—IV, 6. The Worry Diary indicated 23% of the day spent in worry and 92 minutes per day spent in worry. All of these scores were in the normal range. Once treatment has proven effective, the role of the therapist is to prepare the client for continuing the treatment in a self-directed manner.

SELF-DIRECTED CONTINUATION OF TREATMENT

There are four topics to cover when a therapist is preparing a client to continue treatment in a self-directed manner (see Table 9.1): (1) a review of the effective techniques learned in treatment, (2) ways to maintain treatment gains, (3) ways to generalize the treatment to other relevant areas of life, and (4) ways to prevent relapse or handle it if it occurs.

Review of Techniques Learned in Treatment

The review of techniques at the end of treatment will depend upon what has been found effective throughout the course of treatment. The review should include any component that has helped the client reduce the frequency, intensity, and/or duration of worry.

In Richard's case, he found cognitive restructuring (CR), worry exposure, applied relaxation (AR), scheduled worry time, improving problem orientation, response prevention, and pleasurable activity scheduling to be the most effective techniques for reducing his worry. He also found various interpersonal effectiveness techniques helpful for improving his relationships with others at work. These techniques were fully reviewed in the last two treatment sessions.

In these last two sessions, the therapist briefly reviewed the components of the anxiety experience (see Handout 4.1) and related how each of the treatment techniques allowed Richard to make specific changes in each of the components to reduce worry. CR increased Richard's awareness of and ability to challenge cognitive distortions. Worry exposure reduced his avoidance of and emotional reactivity to fearful images. Richard learned how to contain his worry better with scheduled worry time. Improving problem orientation helped him to differentiate the relative significance of various problems and to let go of the worry associated with those that were not key. Richard gained mastery of regulating his physiological arousal with AR. Response prevention and pleasurable activity scheduling allowed him to change behaviors that had been validating and maintaining his worry. Finally (and as noted earlier), to address the problematic patterns of interpersonal interaction that were exacerbating and maintaining some of Richard's symptoms, various techniques for increasing interpersonal effectiveness were employed: assertiveness training, role plays, reversed role plays, reframing the relationship, and exploring links between current and past patterns. These techniques increased Richard's awareness of, and gave him concrete strategies for, altering these patterns of interpersonal behavior.

TABLE 9.1. Agenda for Preparing Client to End Treatment but Continue Skills Practice

1. Review the effective techniques learned.
2. Discuss and plan ways for client to maintain treatment gains.
3. Discuss and plan ways for client to generalize treatment to other relevant life areas.
4. Discuss how to prevent relapse, and plan for what to do if relapses occur.

Maintenance of Treatment Gains

Maintaining the gains made in treatment requires that the client continue practicing the various techniques on a regular basis. An analogy to taking a prescribed medicine can be made: When a person goes to the doctor and receives medication for a certain ailment, the medication is effective only if it is continued for a period of time after the symptoms have been reduced or eliminated. Taking the medication as prescribed by the doctor requires self-discipline. Similarly, the techniques learned in treatment are truly potent only after they have been overpracticed and the lessons from them have been overlearned. The ultimate goal with these techniques is to learn them to such a degree that they become internalized automatic responses, in and of themselves. Disciplining oneself to continue practicing these techniques on a regular basis will ensure that this goal will be met.

In Richard's case, the therapist told Richard that maintaining progress following treatment would require him to continue implementing treatment techniques on a regular basis. The therapist warned Richard about most clients' natural tendency to stop practicing techniques when they are feeling better, and especially when the structure of formal treatment is removed. To counteract this tendency, the therapist discussed with Richard how and when techniques should be practiced after the end of treatment. Throughout this discussion, Richard was queried as to how he might regularly apply the techniques within his daily routine and on weekends and vacations. He was also encouraged to anticipate worrisome situations and ways that he might best cope with those situations. The therapist suggested that Richard regularly schedule a period of time, similar to the time he had set aside for therapy, to do this on a weekly basis. Richard was reminded to use any episode of worry to practice the newly learned techniques, and to continue using the forms as reminders to practice and as self-checks on proper applications. Only when Richard noticed that he was applying techniques in an automatic rather than a deliberate manner, and experiencing the forms simply as redundancies of the practices, could the forms be eliminated.

Generalization of Treatment

The generalization of the treatment to many areas of the client's life is extremely important for a client with GAD. The treatment thus far has provided the client with tools for recognizing and restructuring his or her responses whenever an episode of worry is noticed. In order for the client to maximize the effects of this treatment, it is very important for the client to use these newly learned responses under as many worry-related circumstances as possible. Collaboratively mapping out a step-by-step plan of attack with clearly identified goals (using the graded hierarchies already developed in treatment) will help the client to continue the treatment in a self-directed manner, independently of the therapist.

In Richard's case, the therapist and Richard looked over the hierarchy that had been created in treatment (see Figure 6.1). Richard noticed that he had worked his way through a little over half of the items on this hierarchy. Upon this review, it became clear to both Richard and the therapist that Richard wanted to continue making progress with reducing worry under more circumstances. To accomplish this goal, the therapist encouraged Richard to think about how he might structure and systematically work through the remaining items on the hierarchy after treatment ended. Richard noticed that some of the items on this hierarchy were quite specific and not open for structured practices other than through imagery (e.g., the toilet at home starting to leak, a partner's daughter dying from a serious illness). With these items, Richard thought of other items that would be comparable (e.g., inspecting the house for potential problem areas, reading a medical text about childhood diseases). Richard then described ways that he could set up weekly practices for all of the remaining items, and developed a schedule for these practices (e.g., "Thursday—inspect basement foundation of house for cracks or water leakage; Saturday—inspect house attic for leaks in roof," etc.). The therapist instructed Richard to enter specific practices on his weekly calendar over the course of the next 2 months. The therapist also advised Richard to schedule more practices on his calendar when this period of time ended. Richard committed himself to at least three practices every week, under normal circumstances. He also committed to rescheduling himself after 2 months and to generating new items for the hierarchy.

Relapse Prevention

Preparing the client for the possibility of relapse is essential. The main goal of relapse prevention is to prepare the client to frame relapses as opportunities to learn better ways of coping with such events in the future.

Preparing for situations where a relapse is possible involves three steps. First the client has to identify stimulus events that pose a high risk of relapse. Second, the client has to identify the automatic responses that are likely to be elicited. Third, the client has to identify and plan to use an alternative set of responses to such events. The third step primarily involves the application of techniques already mastered in treatment. Identifying high-risk stimuli requires that the client search both recent and remote memories for events where there have been difficulties with controlling worry. These events may be external and/or internal. The client may find it helpful to draw up a list of those events and similar events anticipated in the future. Preliminary identification of high-risk events and the likely automatic responses can increase awareness when such events are confronted. This in turn assists in the disruption of automatic responding to such events. Identification of high-risk events also allows the client to anticipate and prepare more appropriate cognitive, behavioral, and physiological responses for such circumstances.

Occasionally, clients will underestimate their ability to cope with difficult circumstances following treatment. Clients may have thoughts such as "I can't handle this." These types of thoughts can be challenged with the CR techniques learned in treatment. The therapist and client can prepare a list of rational responses to review under such later circumstances. The following are a few such responses:

- "I've coped with difficult situations before. I can do it again."
- "I can view this as an opportunity to practice what I've learned in treatment."
- "I can use this situation to find out what techniques work best for me."
- "I will succeed in overcoming this with continued effort."

Such statements as these can help the client to maintain hope and motivation despite setbacks. Preparing for relapse also involves increasing the client's awareness of typical cognitive distortions that can follow a relapse, and training the client to identify the reasons for the relapse.

Several types of cognitive distortions may occur following a relapse. Polarized thinking (e.g., "This therapy is useless") may be present. Overgeneralized thinking and jumping to conclusions (e.g., "I'm always going to feel this way") also may be present. Once the client identifies such thoughts, he or she can use the Rational Response Form (Handout 5.4) to challenge such thoughts, and thereby weaken the negative emotional impact of these types of distortions.

Identifying the reasons for a relapse will help the client to regain a sense of control. Assisting the client with reconstructing the chain of events that led up to the relapse can highlight possible areas in need of further therapeutic attention. Imagery techniques can be used to reconstruct the chain of events. Once the problematic points are identified, appropriate responses can be rehearsed for future reference.

Another reason for relapse is that the client experiences difficulty with countering beliefs in the benefits of the old strategies under particularly stressful conditions. In these instances, a cost–benefit analysis of old strategies versus new strategies may help the client to regain his or her motivation to continue breaking old patterns.

Whatever the reason for a relapse, if the client is experiencing renewed difficulties with GAD symptoms following the relapse, he or she should be advised to return for one or more booster sessions for assistance with the implementation of the techniques.

THE IMPORTANCE OF COGNITIVE-BEHAVIORAL THERAPY FOR GAD IN THE EVOLVING HEALTH CARE ENVIRONMENT

Clearly, as discussed in this book, GAD is a widely prevalent, clinically significant syndrome requiring treatment. Several classes of medication (e.g., benzodiazepines such as alprazolam, antidepressants such as venlafaxine) have been shown to be effective for GAD. However, to date, the only psychosocial treatment with proven efficacy is cognitive-behavioral therapy (CBT). The components of this treatment (e.g., CR, relaxation training) are detailed in this book. CBT is not without its limitations, however. This book also presents research on factors that limit the effectiveness of CBT for GAD. Newly developed treatment packages that address these limitations and are currently under investigation are also presented in this book, to inform the clinician of cutting-edge research and researchers in this field. Although continued efforts are being focused on improving treatment, CBT is the best available empirically based psychotherapeutic intervention for GAD at this time.

Disseminating the empirically supported treatment strategies outlined in this book to practitioners in the field is of utmost importance. Consider the following case to illustrate this point. A person with GAD presents to a psychologist for treatment. What type of treatment is he or she likely to receive? More specifically, what is the likelihood that this person will receive the intervention with the most supporting evidence for its efficacy, CBT?

Despite the fact that CBT is the only psychosocial treatment meeting criteria as an empirically supported treatment for GAD (Chambless & Ollendick, 2000), it appears as though only a minority of such patients receive this intervention. Although we know very little about what type of psychological treatments patients actually receive, the existing data suggest that evidence-based treatments are not typically administered (cf. Weissman & Sanderson, 2002). Goisman, Warshaw, and Keller (1999) examined the types of psychosocial treatments received by patients with GAD, panic disorder, and social phobia. The survey was conducted in 1995–1996. Only 34% of these patients reported ever receiving cognitive or behavioral treatments. The investigators found that dynamic psychotherapy was still the most frequently used therapeutic approach. A particularly surprising finding was that the percentage of patients receiving cognitive or behavioral treatments had actually *decreased* from the percentage in a survey conducted by these authors 5 years earlier (1991; Goisman et al., 1993). One would expect an increase—not a decrease—in the use of evidence-based treatments, with the growing body of research and emphasis on evidence-based practice in recent years.

Although these data pertain to the treatment of certain anxiety disorders, there is no reason to suspect that the same situation does not exist for other commonly encountered emotional disorders as well (e.g., major depression, obsessive–compulsive disorder, bulimia nervosa, social phobia). Simply stated, the problem is that there appears to be a gap between those treatments found to be effective in research trials and those practiced in the "real world."

What are the implications of poor dissemination of evidence-based treatments? The poor record of disseminating these treatments from research settings to clinical practitioners in the field has resulted in the lack of availability of many such treatments, as demonstrated by the Goisman et al. (1993, 1999) surveys. This may ultimately have a disastrous impact on the viability of psychotherapy as the health care system evolves (Sanderson, 1997). The increasing penetration of managed care, and the development and proliferation of clinical practice guidelines and treatment consensus statements, have raised the stakes for accountability. The failure to train practitioners in evidence-based treatments may lead to the fall of psychotherapy as a first-line effective treatment, despite considerable data supporting its efficacy. Since managed care organizations and federal guidelines cannot rely on the delivery of treatments that are not widely available, these treatments are often given secondary status, despite their equivalent efficacy (Barlow, 1994). If psychotherapy providers are not trained to provide evidence-based treatments, where do they fall in this new health care scheme? All psychotherapists should be concerned about this issue, because it is paramount to the survival of psychotherapy as a viable treatment. Learning to provide evidence-based treatments, such as the one presented in this book, is essential to keep psychosocial treatments available as first-line treatments for emotional disorders.

References

Alden, L. E., Wiggins, J. S., & Pincus, A. L. (1990). Construction of circumplex scales for the Inventory of Interpersonal Problems. *Journal of Personality Assessment, 55*, 521–536.

Alnaes, R., & Torgersen, S. (1999). A 6-year follow-up study of anxiety disorders in psychiatric outpatients: Development and continuity with personality disorders and personality traits as predictors. *Nordic Journal of Psychiatry, 53*, 409–416.

American Psychiatric Association (APA). (1980). *Diagnostic and statistical manual of mental disorders* (3rd ed.). Washington, DC: Author.

American Psychiatric Association (APA). (1987). *Diagnostic and statistical manual of mental disorders* (3rd ed., rev.). Washington, DC: Author.

American Psychiatric Association (APA). (1994). *Diagnostic and statistical manual of mental disorders* (4th ed.). Washington, DC: Author.

American Psychiatric Association (APA). (2000). *Diagnostic and statistical manual of mental disorders* (4th ed., text rev.). Washington, DC: Author.

Andrews, G., Stewart, G., Allen, R., & Henderson, A. S. (1990). The genetics of six neurotic disorders: A twin study. *Journal of Affective Disorders, 19*, 23–29.

Angst, J., & Vollrath, M. (1991). The natural history of anxiety disorders. *Acta Psychiatrica Scandinavica, 141*, 446–452.

Ballenger, J. C. (1999). Current treatments of the anxiety disorders in adults. *Biological Psychiatry, 46*, 1579–1594.

Ballenger, J. C., Davidson, J. R. T., Lecrubier, Y., Nutt, D. J., Borkovec, T. D., Rickels, K., et al. (2001). Consensus statement on generalized anxiety disorder from the International Consensus Group on Depression and Anxiety. *Journal of Clinical Psychiatry, 62*, 53–58.

Barlow, D. H. (1994). Psychological interventions in the era of managed care. *Clinical Psychology: Science and Practice, 1*, 109–122.

Barlow, D. H. (2002). *Anxiety and its disorders: The nature and treatment of anxiety and panic* (2nd ed.). New York: Guilford Press.

Barlow, D. H., Cohen, A. S., Waddell, M. T., Vermilyea, B. B., Klosko, J. S., Blanchard, E. B., et al. (1984). Panic and generalized anxiety disorders: Nature and treatment. *Behavior Therapy, 15*, 431–449.

Barlow, D. H., Rapee, R. M., & Brown, T. A. (1992). Treatment of generalized anxiety disorder. *Behavior Therapy, 23*, 552–582.

Barman Balfour, J. A., & Jarvis, B. (2000). Venlafaxine extended-release: A review of its clinical potential in the management of generalized anxiety disorder. *CNS Drugs, 14,* 483–503.

Beck, A. T., & Emery, G., with Greenberg, R. L. (1985). *Anxiety disorders and phobias: A cognitive perspective.* New York: Basic Books.

Beck, A. T., Epstein, N., Brown, G., & Steer, R. A. (1988). An inventory for measuring clinical anxiety: Psychometric properties. *Journal of Consulting and Clinical Psychology, 56,* 893–897.

Beck, A. T., Steer, R. A., & Brown, G. K. (1996). *Beck Depression Inventory manual* (2nd ed.). San Antonio, TX: Psychological Corporation.

Ben-Noun, L. (1998). Generalized anxiety disorder in dysfunctional families. *Journal of Behavior Therapy and Experimental Psychiatry, 29,* 115–122.

Bland, R. C., Newman, S. C., & Orn, H. (1997). Help-seeking for psychiatric disorders. *Canadian Journal of Psychiatry, 42,* 935–942.

Blazer, D. G., George, L. K., & Hughes, D. (1991). The epidemiology of anxiety disorders: An age comparison. In C. Salzman & B. D. Lebowitz (Eds.), *Anxiety in the elderly: Treatment and research* (pp. 17–30). New York: Springer.

Blowers, C., Cobb, J., & Mathews, A. (1987). generalized anxiety: A controlled treatment study. *Behaviour Research and Therapy, 25,* 493–502.

Borkovec, T. D. (1979). Extension of two-factor theory: Cognitive avoidance and autonomic perception. In N. Birbaumer & H. D. Kimmel (Eds.), *Biofeedback and self-regulation* (pp. 139–148). Hillsdale, NJ: Erlbaum.

Borkovec, T. D. (1994). The nature, functions, and origins of worry. In G. C. L. Davey & F. Tallis (Eds.), *Worrying: Perspectives on theory, assessment, and treatment* (pp. 5–33). Chichester, England: Wiley.

Borkovec, T. D., Alcaine, O. M., & Behar, E. (2004). Avoidance theory of worry and generalized anxiety disorder. In R. G. Heimberg, C. L. Turk, & D. S. Mennin (Eds.), *Generalized anxiety disorder: Advances in research and practice* (pp. 77–108). New York: Guilford Press.

Borkovec, T. D., & Costello, E. (1993). Efficacy of applied relaxation and cognitive behavioral therapy in the treatment of generalized anxiety disorder. *Journal of Consulting and Clinical Psychology, 61,* 611–619.

Borkovec. T. D., & Inz, J. (1990). The nature of worry in generalized anxiety disorder: A predominance of thought activity. *Behaviour Research and Therapy, 28,* 153–158.

Borkovec, T. D., & Mathews, A. M. (1988). Treatment of nonphobic anxiety disorders: A comparison of nondirective, cognitive, and coping desensitization therapy. *Journal of Consulting and Clinical Psychology, 56,* 877–884.

Borkovec, T. D., Mathews, A. M., Chambers, A., Ebrahimi, S., Lytle, R., & Nelson, R. (1987). The effects of relaxation training with cognitive or nondirective therapy and the role of relaxation-induced anxiety in the treatment of generalized anxiety. *Journal of Consulting and Clinical Psychology, 55,* 883–888.

Borkovec, T. D., Newman, M. G., Pincus, A. L., & Lytle, R. (2002). A component analysis of cognitive behavioral therapy for generalized anxiety disorder and the role of interpersonal problems. *Journal of Consulting and Clinical Psychology, 70,* 288–298.

Borkovec, T. D., & Roemer, L. (1994). Generalized anxiety disorder. In M. Hersen & R. T. Ammerman (Eds.), *Handbook of prescriptive treatments for adults* (pp. 261–281). New York: Plenum Press.

Borkovec, T. D., & Roemer, L. (1995). Perceived functions of worry among generalized anxiety disorder subjects: Distraction from more emotional topics? *Journal of Behavior Therapy and Experimental Psychiatry, 26,* 25–30.

Borkovec, T. D., & Ruscio, A. M. (2001). Psychotherapy for generalized anxiety disorder. *Journal of Consulting and Clinical Psychology, 62,* 37–42.

Borkovec, T. D., & Whisman, M. A. (1996). Psychological treatment for generalized anxiety disorder. In M. R. Mavissakalian & R. F. Prien (Eds.), *Long-term treatments of anxiety disorders* (pp. 171–199). Washington, DC: American Psychiatric Press.

Borkovec, T. D., Wilkinson, L., Folensbee, R., & Lerman, C. (1983). Stimulus control applications to the treatment of worry. *Behaviour Research and Therapy, 21,* 247–251.

Brawman-Mintzer, O., & Lydiard, R. B. (1996). Biological basis of generalized anxiety disorder. *Journal of Clinical Psychiatry, 58,* 16–25.

Brown, T. A., Antony, M. M., & Barlow, D. H. (1992). Psychometric properties of the Penn State Worry Questionnaire in a clinical anxiety disorders sample. *Behaviour Research and Therapy, 30,* 33–37.

Brown, T. A., & Barlow, D. H. (1992). Comorbidity among anxiety disorders: Implications for treatment and DSM-IV. *Journal of Consulting and Clinical Psychology, 60,* 835–844.

Brown, T. A., Moras, K., Zinberg, R. E., & Barlow, D. H. (1993). Diagnostic and symptom distinguishability of generalized anxiety disorder and obsessive–compulsive disorder. *Behavior Therapy, 24,* 227–240.

Burns, D. D. (1980). *Feeling good: The new mood therapy.* New York: Morrow.

Butler, G., Cullington, A., Hibbert, G., Klimes, I., & Gelder, M. (1987). Anxiety management for persistent generalized anxiety. *British Journal of Psychiatry, 151,* 535–542.

Butler, G., Fennell, M., Robson, P., & Gelder, M. (1991). Comparison of behavior therapy and cognitive behavior therapy in the treatment of generalized anxiety disorder. *Journal of Consulting and Clinical Psychology, 59,* 167–175.

Carter, R. M., Wittchen, H.-U., Pfister, H., & Kessler, R. C. (2001). One-year prevalence of subthreshold and threshold DSM-IV generalized anxiety disorder in a nationally representative sample. *Depression and Anxiety, 13,* 78–88.

Chambless, D. L., & Gillis, M. M. (1993). Cognitive therapy of anxiety disorders. *Journal of Consulting and Clinical Psychology, 61,* 248–260.

Chambless, D. L., & Ollendick, T. H. (2000). Empirically supported psychological interventions: Controversies and evidence. *Annual Review of Psychology, 52,* 685–716.

Chorpita, B. F., & Barlow, D. H. (1998). The development of anxiety: The role of control in the early environment. *Psychological Bulletin, 124,* 3–21.

Clark, D. M., Ball, S., & Pape, D. (1991). An experimental investigation of thought suppression. *Behaviour Research and Therapy, 29,* 253–257.

Clark, D. M., Salkovskis, P., & Chalkley, A. (1985). Respiratory control as a treatment for panic attacks. *Journal of Behavior Therapy and Experimental Psychiatry, 16,* 23–30.

Clark, L. A., Watson, D., & Mineka, S. (1994). Temperament, personality, and the mood and anxiety disorders. *Journal of Abnormal Psychology, 103,* 103–116.

Craske, M. G., Barlow, D. H., & O'Leary, T. A. (1992). *Mastery of your anxiety and worry: Client workbook.* Albany, NY: Graywind.

Craske, M. G., & Hazlett-Stevens, H. (2002). Facilitating symptom reduction and behavior change in GAD: The issue of control. *Clinical Psychology: Science and Practice, 9,* 69–75.

Craske, M. G., Rapee, R. M., Jackel, L., & Barlow, D. H. (1989). Qualitative dimensions of worry in DSM-III-R generalized anxiety disorder subjects and nonanxious controls. *Behaviour Research and Therapy, 27,* 397–402.

Davey, G. C. L. (1994a). Pathological worrying as exacerbated problem solving. In G. C. L. Davey & F. Tallis (Eds.), *Worrying: Perspectives on theory, assessment, and treatment* (pp. 35–59). Chichester, England: Wiley.

Davey, G. C. L. (1994b). Worrying, social problem-solving abilities, and social problem-solving confidence. *Behaviour Research and Therapy, 32,* 327–330.

Davey, G. C. L., Hampton, J., Farrell, J. L., & Davidson, S. (1992). Some characteristics of worrying: Evidence for worrying and anxiety as separate constructs. *Personality and Individual Differences, 13,* 133–147.

Davidson, J. R. T., DuPont, R. L., Hedges, D., & Haskins, J. T. (1999). Efficacy, safety, and tolerability of venlafaxine extended release and buspirone in outpatients with generalized anxiety disorder: A 6-month randomized control trial. *Journal of Clinical Psychiatry, 60,* 528–535.

Davis, R. N., & Valentiner, D. P. (2000). Does meta-cognitive theory enhance our understanding of pathological worry and anxiety? *Personality and Individual Differences, 29,* 513–526.

DiNardo, P. A., Brown, T. A., & Barlow, D. H. (1994). *Anxiety Disorders Interview Schedule for DSM-IV.* Boston: Center for Stress and Anxiety Related Disorders, Boston University.

Dugas, M. J., Gagnon, F., Ladouceur, R., & Freeston, M. H. (1998). Generalized anxiety disorder: A preliminary test of a conceptual model. *Behaviour Research and Therapy, 36,* 215–226.

Dupuy, J. B., Beaudoin, S., Rheaume, J., Ladouceur, R., & Dugas, M. J. (2001). Worry: Daily self-report in clinical and non-clinical populations. *Behaviour Research and Therapy, 39,* 1249–1255.

Durham, R. C., Allan, T., & Hackett, C. A. (1997). On predicting improvement and relapse in generalized anxiety disorder following psychotherapy. *British Journal of Clinical Psychology, 36,* 101–119.

Durham, R. C., Fisher, P. L., Treliving, L. R., Hau, C. M., Richard, K., & Stewart, J. B. (1999). One year follow-up of cognitive therapy, analytic psychotherapy and anxiety management training for generalized anxiety disorder: Symptom change, medication usage and attitudes to treatment. *Behavioural and Cognitive Psychotherapy, 27,* 19–35.

Durham, R. C., Murphy, T., Allan, T., Richard, K., Treliving, L. R., & Fenton, G. W. (1994). Cognitive therapy, analytic psychotherapy and anxiety management training for generalized anxiety disorder. *British Journal of Psychiatry, 165,* 315–323.

Durham, R. C., & Turvey, A. A. (1987). Cognitive therapy vs. behaviour therapy in the treatment of chronic generalized anxiety. *Behaviour Research and Therapy, 25,* 229–234.

Dyck, I. R., Phillips, K. A., Warshaw, M. G., Dolan, R. T., Shea, M. T., Stout, R. L., et al. (2001). Patterns of personality pathology in patients with generalized anxiety disorder, panic disorder with and without agoraphobia, and social phobia. *Journal of Personality Disorders, 15,* 60–71.

El-Khayat, R., & Baldwin, D. S. (1998). Antipsychotic drugs for non-psychotic patients: Assessment of the benefit/risk ratio in generalized anxiety disorder. *Journal of Psychopharmacology, 12,* 323–329.

Finlay-Jones, R., & Brown, G. W. (1981). Types of stressful life events and the onset of anxiety and depressive disorders. *Psychological Medicine, 11,* 803–815.

First, M. B., Spitzer, R. L., Gibbon, M., & Williams, J. B. (1996). *Structured Clinical Interview for DSM-IV Axis I Disorders, Clinical Version (SCID-CV).* Washington, DC: American Psychiatric Press.

First, M. B., Spitzer, R. L., Gibbon, M., & Williams, J. B. (1997). *Structured Clinical Interview for DSM-IV Personality Disorder (SCID-II).* Washington, DC: American Psychiatric Press.

Fisher, P. L., & Durham, R. C. (1999). Recovery rates in generalized anxiety disorder following psychological therapy: An analysis of clinically significant change in the STAI-T across outcome studies since 1990. *Psychological Medicine, 29,* 1425–1434.

Foa, E. B., & Kozak, M. J. (1986). Emotional processing of fear: Exposure to corrective information. *Psychological Bulletin, 99,* 20–35.

Follette, V. M. (1994). Survivors of child sexual abuse: Treatment using a contextual analysis. In S. C. Hayes, N. S. Jacobson, V. M. Follette, & M. J. Dougher (Eds.), *Acceptance and change: Content and context in psychotherapy* (pp. 255–268). Reno, NV: Context Press.

Freeston, M. H., Rheaume, J., Letarte, H., Dugas, M. J., & Ladouceur, R. (1994). Why do people worry? *Personality and Individual Differences, 17,* 791–802.

Gershuny, B. S., & Sher, K. J. (1998). The relation between personality and anxiety: Findings from a 3-year prospective study. *Journal of Abnormal Psychology, 107,* 252–262.

Goisman, R. M., Rogers, M. P., Steketee, G. S., Warshaw, M. G., Cuneo, P., & Keller, M. B. (1993). Utilization of behavioral methods in a multi-center anxiety disorders study. *Journal of Clinical Psychiatry, 54,* 213–218.

Goisman, R. M., Warshaw, M. G., & Keller, M. B. (1999). Psychosocial treatment prescriptions for generalized anxiety disorder, panic disorder, and social phobia, 1991–1996. *American Journal of Psychiatry, 156,* 1819–1821.

Goldfried, M. R. (1971). Systematic desensitization as training in self-control. *Journal of Consulting and Clinical Psychology, 37,* 228–234.

Gould, R. A., Otto, M. W., Pollack, M. H., & Yap, L. (1997). Cognitive behavioral and pharmacological treatment of generalized anxiety disorder: A preliminary meta-analysis. *Behavior Therapy, 28,* 285–305.

Greenberg, L. S., & Safran, J. D. (1987). *Emotion in psychotherapy*. New York: Guilford Press.

Greenberg, P. E., Sisitsky, T., Kessler, R. C., Finkelstein, S. N., Berndt, E. R., Davidson, J. R. T., et al. (1999). The economic burden of the anxiety disorders in the 1990s. *Journal of Clinical Psychiatry, 60,* 427–435.

Harvey, A. G., & Rapee, R. M. (1995). Cognitive-behavior therapy for generalized anxiety disorder. *Psychiatric Clinics of North America, 18,* 859–870.

Hayes, S. C., Strosahl, K. D., & Wilson, K. G. (1999). *Acceptance and commitment therapy: An experiential approach to behavior change*. New York: Guilford Press.

Hettema, J. M., Prescott, C. A., & Kendler, K. S. (2001). A population-based twin study of generalized anxiety disorder in men and women. *Journal of Nervous and Mental Disease, 189,* 413–420.

Hudson, J. L., & Rapee, R. M. (2004). From anxious temperament to disorder: An etiological model of generalized anxiety disorder. In R. G. Heimberg, C. L. Turk, & D. S. Mennin (Eds.), *Generalized anxiety disorder: Advances in research and practice* (pp. 51–74). New York: Guilford Press.

Jacobson, E. (1929). *Progressive relaxation*. Chicago, IL: University of Chicago Press.

Kabat-Zinn, J. (1990). *Full catastrophic living: Using the wisdom of your body and mind to face stress, pain, and illness*. New York: Delacorte Press.

Kendler, K. S., Neale, M. C., Kessler, R. C., Heath, A. C., & Eaves, L. J. (1992). Major depression and generalized anxiety disorder: Same genes, (partly) different environments? *Archives of General Psychiatry, 49,* 716–722.

Kendler, K. S., Walters, E. E., Neale, M. C., Kessler, R. C., Heath, A. C., & Eaves, L. J. (1995). The structure of the genetic environmental risk factors for six major psychiatric disorders in women: Phobia, generalized anxiety disorder, panic disorder, bulimia, major depression, and alcoholism. *Archives of General Psychiatry, 52,* 374–383.

Kennedy, B. L., & Schwab, J. J. (1997). Utilization of medical specialists by anxiety disorder patients. *Psychosomatics, 38,* 109–1112.

Kessler, R. C. (2000). Gender differences in major depression: Epidemiological findings. In E. Frank (Ed.), *Gender and its effects on psychopathology* (pp. 61–84). Washington, DC: American Psychiatric Press.

Kessler, R. C., DuPont, R. L., Bergllund, P., & Wittchen, H.-U. (1999). Impairment in pure and comorbid generalized anxiety disorder at 12 months in two national surveys. *American Journal of Psychiatry, 156,* 1663–1678.

Kessler, R. C., McGonagle, K. A., Zhao, S., Nelson, C. B., Hughes, M., Eshleman, S., et al. (1994). Lifetime and 12–month prevalence of DSM-III-R psychiatric disorders in the United States: Results from the National Comorbidity Survey. *Archives of General Psychiatry, 51,* 8–19.

Klosko, J. S., & Sanderson, W. C. (1999). *Cognitive-behavioral treatment of depression*. Northvale, NJ: Jason Aronson.

Ladouceur, R., Blais, F., Freeston, M. H., & Dugas, M. J. (1998). Problem solving and problem orientation in generalized anxiety disorder. *Journal of Anxiety Disorders, 12,* 139–152.

Ladouceur, R., Dugas, M. J., Freeston, M. H., Leger, E., Gagnon, F., & Thibodeau, N. (2000). Efficacy of a new cognitive-behavioral treatment for generalized anxiety disorder: Evaluation in a controlled clinical trial. *Journal of Consulting and Clinical Psychology, 68,* 957–964.

Ladouceur, R., Talbot, F., & Dugas, M. J. (1997). Behavioral expressions of intolerance of uncertainty in worry: Experimental findings. *Behavior Modification, 21,* 355–371.

Lang, P. J. (1978). Anxiety: Toward a psychophysiological definition. In H. S. Akiskal & W. L. Webb (Eds.), *Psychiatric diagnosis: Exploration of biological predictors* (pp. 365–389). New York: Spectrum.

Lang, P. J. (1979). A bio-informational theory of emotional imagery. *Psychophysiology, 16,* 495–512.

Lang, P. J. (1985). The cognitive psychophysiology of emotion: Fear and anxiety. In A. H. Tuma & J. D. Maser (Eds.), *Anxiety and the anxiety disorders* (pp. 131–170). Hillsdale, NJ: Erlbaum.

Lang, P. J. (1994). Varieties of emotional experience: A mediation on James–Lange theory. *Psychological Review, 101,* 211–221.

Lang, P. J., Cuthbert, B. N., & Bradley, M. M. (1998). Measuring emotion in therapy: Imagery, activation, and feeling. *Behavior Therapy, 29,* 655–674.

Lewinsohn, P. M. (1975). The behavioral study and treatment of depression. In M. Hersen & R. M. Eisler (Eds.), *Progress in behavior modification* (pp. 19–64). New York: Academic Press.

Lichtenstein, J., & Cassidy, J. (1991, April). *The Inventory of Adult Attachment (INVAA): Validation of a new measure.* Paper presented at the biennial meeting of the Society for Research in Child Development, Seattle, WA.

Lindsay, W. R., Gamsu, C. V., McLaughlin, F., Hood, E., & Espie, C. A. (1987). A controlled trial of treatments for generalized anxiety. *British Journal of Clinical Psychology, 26,* 3–15.

Linehan, M. M. (1993a). *Cognitive-behavioral treatment of borderline personality disorder.* New York: Guilford Press.

Linehan, M. M. (1993b). *Skills training manual for treating borderline personality disorder.* New York: Guilford Press.

Mahe, V., & Balogh, A. (2000). Long-term pharmacological treatment of generalized anxiety disorder. *International Clinical Psychopharmacology, 15,* 99–105.

Mancuso, D. M., Townsend, M. H., & Mercante, D. E. (1993). Long-term follow-up of generalized anxiety disorder. *Comprehensive Psychiatry, 34,* 441–446.

Martinsen, E. W., Sandvik, L., & Kolbjornsrud, O.-B. (1989). Aerobic exercise in the treatment of nonpsychotic mental disorders: An explanatory study. *Nordisk Psykiatrisk Tidsskrift, 43,* 521–529.

Mavissakalian, M. R., Hamann, M. S., Haidaar, S. A., & De Groot, C. M. (1995). Correlates of DSM-III personality disorder in generalized anxiety disorder. *Journal of Anxiety Disorders, 9,* 103–115.

Mennin, D. S., Heimberg, R. G., Turk, C. L., & Fresco, D. M. (2002). Applying an emotion regulation framework to integrative approaches to generalized anxiety disorder. *Clinical Psychology: Science and Practice, 9,* 85–90.

Meoni, P., Salinas, E., Brault, Y., & Hackett, D. (2001). Pattern of symptom improvement following treatment with venlafaxine XR in patients with generalized anxiety disorder. *Journal of Clinical Psychiatry, 62,* 888–893.

Meyer, T. J., Miller, M. L., Metzger, R. L., & Borkovec, T. D. (1990). Development and validation of the Penn State Worry Questionnaire. *Behaviour Research and Therapy, 28,* 487–495.

Molina, S., & Borkovec, T. D. (1994). The Penn State Worry Questionnaire: Psychometric properties and associated characteristics. In G. C. Davey & F. Tallis (Eds.), *Worrying: Perspectives on theory, assessment, and treatment* (pp. 265–283). Chichester, England: Wiley.

Mowrer, O. H. (1947). On the dual nature of learning: A re-interpretation of "conditioning" and "problem solving." *Harvard Educational Review, 17,* 102–148.

Newman, M. G. (2000). Recommendations for a cost offset model of psychotherapy allocation using generalized anxiety disorder as an example. *Journal of Consulting and Clinical Psychology, 68,* 549–555.

Newman, M. G., Castonguay, L. G., Borkovec, T. D., & Molnar, C. (2004). Integrative psychotherapy. In R. G. Heimberg, C. L. Turk, & D. S. Mennin (Eds.), *Generalized anxiety disorder: Advances in research and practice* (pp. 320–350). New York: Guilford Press.

Newman, M. G., Zuellig, A. R., Kachin, K. E., Constantino, M. J., Przeworski, A., Erikson, T., et al. (2002). Preliminary reliability and validity of the Generalized Anxiety Disorder Questionnaire—IV: A revised self-report diagnostic measure of generalized anxiety disorder. *Behavior Therapy, 33,* 215–233.

Noyes, R., Woodman, C., Garvey, M. J., Cook, B. L., Suelzer, M., Chancy, J., et al. (1992). Generalized anxiety disorder vs. panic disorder: Distinguishing characteristics and patterns of comorbidity. *Journal of Nervous and Mental Disease, 180,* 369–379.

Ormel, J., Von Korff, M., Ustun, B., Pini, S., Korten, A., & Oldehinkel, T. (1994). Common mental disorders and disabilities across cultures: Results from the WHO collaborative study on psychological problems in general health care. *Journal of the American Medical Association, 272,* 1741–1748.

Orsillo, S. M., Roemer, L., & Barlow, D. H. (2003). Integrating acceptance and mindfuless into existing cognitive-behavioral treatment for GAD: A case study. *Cognitive and Behavioral Practice, 10,* 223–230.

Öst, L.-G. (1987). Applied relaxation: Description of a coping technique and review of controlled studies. *Behaviour Research and Therapy, 25,* 397–409.

Öst, L.-G., & Breitholtz, E. (2000). Applied relaxation vs. cognitive therapy in the treatment of generalized anxiety disorder. *Behaviour Research and Therapy, 38,* 777–790.

Rapee, R. M. (1991). Generalized anxiety disorder: A review of clinical features and theoretical concepts. *Clinical Psychology Review, 11,* 419–440.

Rickels, K., DeMartinis, N., Garcia-Espana, F., Greenblatt, D. J., Mandas, L. A., & Rynn, M. (2000). Imipramine and buspirone in treatment of patients with generalized anxiety disorder who are discontinuing long-term benzodiazepine therapy. *American Journal of Psychiatry, 157,* 1973–1979.

Rickels, K., Pollack, M. H., Sheehan, D. V., & Haskins, J. T. (2000). Efficacy of extended-release venlafaxine in nondepressed outpatients with generalized anxiety disorder. *American Journal of Psychiatry, 157,* 968–981.

Roemer, L., & Orsillo, S. M. (2002). Expanding our conceptualization of and treatment for generalized anxiety disorder: Integrating mindfulness/acceptance-based approaches with existing cognitive-behavioral models. *Clinical Psychology: Science and Practice, 9,* 54–68.

Sanderson, K., & Andrews, G. (2002). Prevalence and severity of mental-health-related disability and relationship to diagnosis. *Psychiatric Services, 53,* 80–86.

Sanderson, W. C. (1997). The importance of empirically supported psychological interventions in the new healthcare environment. In L. VandeCreek, S. Knapp, & T. Jackson (Eds.), *Innovations in clinical practice: A source book* (Vol. 15, pp. 387–399). Sarasota, FL: Professional Resource Press.

Sanderson, W. C., & Barlow, D. H. (1990). A description of patients diagnosed with DSM-III-R generalized anxiety disorder. *Journal of Nervous and Mental Disease, 178,* 588–591.

Sanderson, W. C., Beck, A. T., & McGinn, L. K. (1994). Cognitive therapy for generalized anxiety disorder: Significance of comorbid personality disorders. *Journal of Cognitive Psychotherapy: An International Quarterly, 8,* 13–18.

Sanderson, W. C., DiNardo, P. A., Rapee, R. M., & Barlow, D. H. (1990). Syndrome comorbidity in patients diagnosed with a DSM-III-Revised anxiety disorder. *Journal of Abnormal Psychology, 99,* 308–312.

Sanderson, W. C., & Wetzler, S. (1991). Chronic anxiety and generalized anxiety disorder: Issues in comorbidity. In R. M. Rapee & D. H. Barlow (Eds.), *Chronic anxiety: Generalized anxiety disorder and mixed anxiety–depression* (pp. 119–135). New York: Guilford Press.

Schatzberg, A. F., Cole, J. O., & DeBattista, C. (1997). *Manual of clinical psychopharmacology* (3rd ed). Washington, DC: American Psychiatric Press.

Schut, A. J., Castonguay, L. G., & Borkovec, T. D. (2001). Compulsive checking behaviors in generalized anxiety disorder. *Journal of Clinical Psychology, 57,* 705–715.

Schweizer, E., & Rickels, K. (1996). The long-term management of generalized anxiety disorder: Issues and dilemmas. *Journal of Clinical Psychiatry, 57,* 9–12.

Schweizer, E., & Rickels, K. (1997). Strategies for treatment of generalized anxiety in the primary care setting. *Journal of Clinical Psychiatry, 58,* 27–31.

Segal, Z. V., Williams, J. M. G., & Teasdale, J. D. (2002). *Mindfulness-based cognitive therapy for depression.* New York: Guilford Press.

Sime, W. (1996). Guidelines for clinical applications of exercise therapy for mental health. In J. L. Van Raalte & B. W. Brewer (Eds.), *Exploring sport and exercise psychology* (pp. 159–187). Washington, DC: American Psychological Association.

Stein, D. J. (2001). Comorbidity in generalized anxiety disorder: Impact and implications. *Journal of Clinical Psychiatry, 62,* 29–36.

Steer, R. A., Brown, G. K., Beck, A. T., & Sanderson, W. C. (1999). Mean Beck Depression Inventory-II scores by severity of major depressive episode. *Psychological Reports, 88,* 1075–1076.

Steer, R. A., Clark, D. A., Beck, A. T., & Ranieri, W. F. (1999). Common and specific dimensions of self-reported anxiety and depression: The BDI-II versus the BDI-IA. *Behaviour Research and Therapy, 37,* 183–190.

Stober, J. (1998). Worry, problem elaboration and suppression of imagery: The role of concreteness. *Behaviour Research and Therapy, 36,* 751–756.

Stober, J., & Borkovec, T. D. (2002). Reduced concreteness of worry in generalized anxiety disorder: Findings from a therapy study. *Cognitive Therapy and Research, 26,* 89–96.

Stober, J., & Joorman, J. (2001). Worry, procrastination, and perfectionism: Differentiating amount of worry, pathological worry, anxiety, and depression. *Cognitive Therapy and Research, 25,* 49–60.

Sussman, N., & Stein, D. J. (2001). Pharmacotherapy for generalized anxiety disorder. In D. Stein & E. Hollander (Eds.), *The American Psychiatric Publishing textbook of anxiety disorders* (pp. 135–140). Washington, DC:American Psychiatric Press.

Teasdale, J. D., Segal, Z. V., Williams, J. M. G., Ridgeway, V. A., Soulsby, J. M., & Lau, M. A. (2000). Prevention of relapse/recurrence in major depression by mindfulness-based cognitive therapy. *Journal of Consulting and Clinical Psychology, 68,* 615–623.

Tkachuk, G. A., & Martin, G. L. (1999). Exercise therapy for patients with psychiatric disorders: Research and clinical implications. *Professional Psychology: Research and Practice, 30,* 275–282.

Trull, T. J., & Sher, K. J. (1994). Relationship between the five-factor model of personality and Axis I disorders in a nonclinical sample. *Journal of Abnormal Psychology, 103,* 350–360.

Vasey, M. W., & Borkovec, T. D. (1992). A catastrophizing assessment of worrisome thoughts. *Cognitive Therapy and Research, 16,* 505–520.

Wegner, D., Schneider, D., Carter, S., & White, T. (1987). Paradoxical effects of thought suppression. *Journal of Personality and Social Psychology, 53,* 5–13.

Weissman, M. M., & Merikangas, K. R. (1986). The epidemiology of anxiety and panic disorders: An update. *Journal of Clinical Psychopharmacology, 46,* 11–17.

Weissman, M. M., & Sanderson, W. C. (2002). Problems and promises in modern psychotherapy: The need for increased training in evidence based treatments. In B. Hamburg (Ed.), *Modern psychiatry: Challenges in educating health professionals to meet new needs.* New York: Josiah Macy Foundation.

Wells, A. (1995). Meta-cognition and worry: A cognitive model of generalized anxiety disorder. *Behavioural and Cognitive Psychotherapy, 23,* 301–320.

Wells, A. (1999). A cognitive model of generalized anxiety disorder. *Behavior Modification, 23,* 526–555.

Wells, A. (2002). GAD, metacognition, and mindfulness: An information processing analysis. *Clinical Psychology: Science and Practice, 9,* 179–192.

White, J. (1998). "Stress control" large group therapy for generalized anxiety disorder: Two year follow-up. *Behavioural and Cognitive Psychotherapy, 26,* 237–245.

White, J., Keenan, M., & Brooks, N. (1992). Stress control: A controlled comparative investigation of large group therapy for generalized anxiety disorder. *Behavioural and Cognitive Psychotherapy, 20,* 97–114.

Wittchen, H.-U., Carter, R. M., Pfister, H., Montgomery, S. A., & Kessler, R. C. (2000). Disabilities and quality of life in pure and comorbid generalized anxiety disorder and major depression in a national survey. *International Clinical Psychopharmacology, 15,* 319–328.

Wittchen, H.-U., Zhao, S., Kessler, R., & Eaton, W. W. (1994). DSM-II-R generalized anxiety disorder in the National Comorbidity Survey. *Archives of General Psychiatry, 51,* 355–364.

Wolpe, J. (1958). *Psychotherapy by reciprocal inhibition.* Stanford, CA: Stanford University Press.

Yonkers, K. A., Dyck, I. R., Warshaw, M., & Keller, M. B. (2000). Factors predicting the clinical course of generalized anxiety disorder. *British Journal of Psychiatry, 176,* 544–549.

Yonkers, K. A., Warshaw, M. G., Massion, A. O., & Keller, M. B. (1996). Phenomenology and course of generalized anxiety disorder. *British Journal of Psychiatry, 168,* 308–313.

Young, J. E., & Klosko, J. S. (1993). *Reinventing your life: How to break free from negative life patterns.* New York: Dutton.

Young, J. E., Klosko, J. S., & Weishaar, M. E. (2003). *Schema therapy: A practitioner's guide.* New York: Guilford Press.

Zinbarg, R. E., Craske, M. G., & Barlow, D. H. (1993). *Mastery of your anxiety and worry: Therapist guide.* Albany, NY: Graywind.

Index